What do vegans eat?

Book Details

Epicentre Equilibrium Publishing

Copyright © 2012 by Leigh-Chantelle
Cover and Design by Adele Walker (www.adelewalker.blogspot.com)
Photographs of Leigh-Chantelle © Adele Walker
Food Photographs © *Viva la Vegan!* & Leigh-Chantelle
Author Portrait by Carol Slater Photography (www.c-s-p.com.au)
Lettering: Leigh-Chantelle

All rights reserved

ISBN 978-0-9808484-0-3

www.epicentreequilibrium.com

Creative Commons: Attribution Non-commercial No Derivatives
http://creativecommons.org/licenses/by-nc-nd/3.0/au

About the Book

Viva la Vegan! started as a scrapbook-style presentation for a Brisbane vegan group in Australia, *Vegan Existence (V.EX)*. I wanted my presentation to be fun and visually appealing, yet still have the important educational aspects of a vegan health talk. I combined my love for fun, easy to comprehend education, with food and animal photographs and myself posing to create what I hope is an inspiring look at how easy being a vegan is in this day. The presentation I gave was around 60 minutes long and there is also a short 5 minute recap video on my YouTube channel (www.youtube.com/vivalavegandotnet).

While I focus mostly on the food aspects of veganism in *What Do Vegans Eat*, I must point out that veganism is not just a diet. Being vegan is a lifestyle and a set of ethical values that myself and many others choose to embrace. I hope that I inspire others by leading by example to show how easy it is to live in line with your ethics and values. I therefore encourage all vegans and potential vegans to educate themselves to the other benefits of the vegan lifestyle. These include: Animal rights and Welfare, Environment and Sustainability, Ethical and moral issues, Health, Spiritual and/or Religious beliefs, Weight loss or control.

Please see my website vivalavegan.net for more information, recipes and to get involved with the vegan revolution.

This is all for the voiceless.

Enjoy,

Leigh-Chantelle

Hi! I'm Leigh-Chantelle

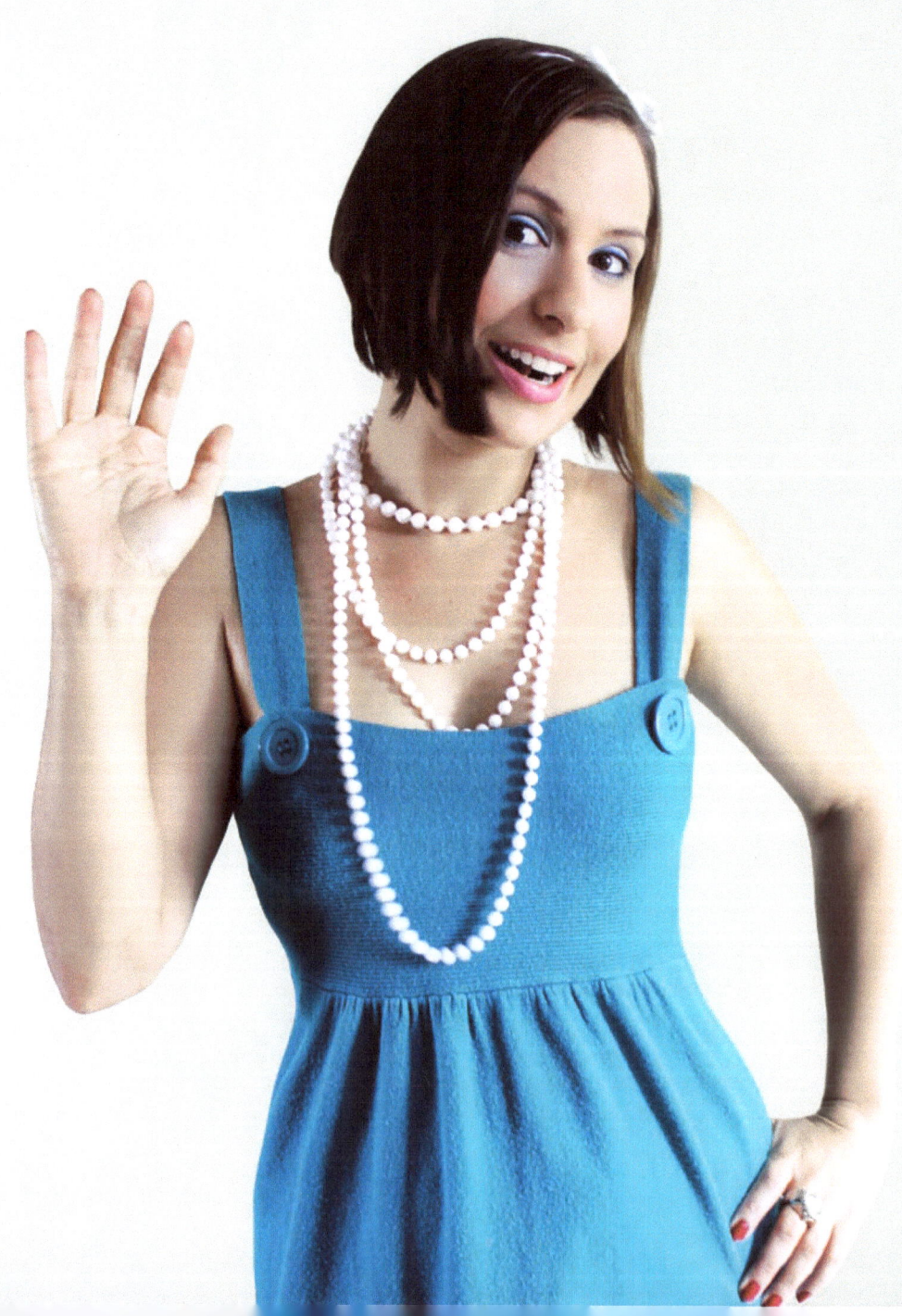

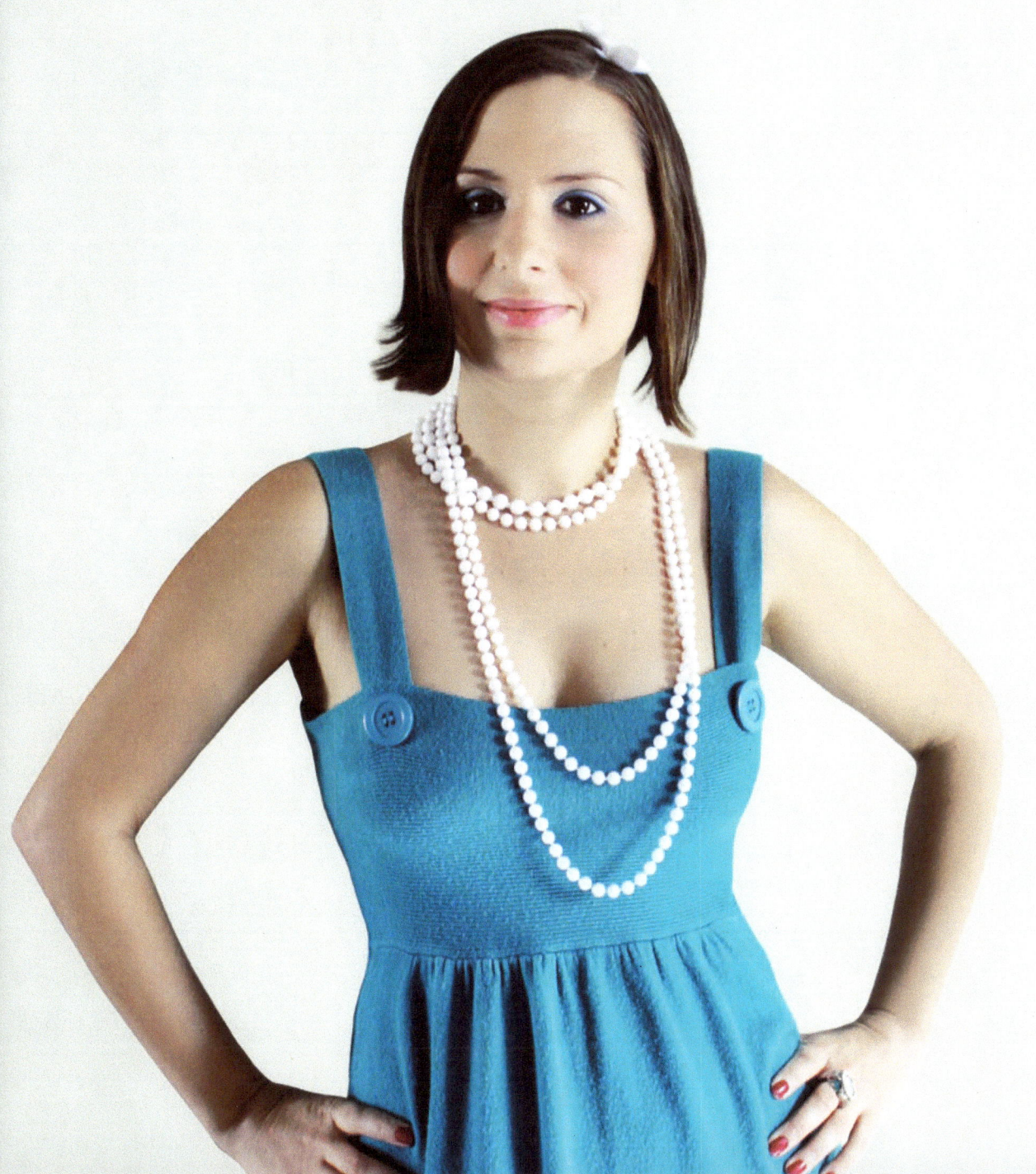

A vegan is a strict vegetarian. <u>No</u> animal products or animal by-products for food, clothing or other purposes.

Incase you don't know, a Vegan is a strict vegetarian who chooses not to consume ANY animal products or by-products for food, clothing or other purposes. This means that vegans choose not eat any animals including chickens and fishes. Vegans choose not consume any animal products or by-products for example milk, honey, eggs, gelatine as well as choosing not to wear leather, fur, silk or wool.

Vegans aim to do their part to stop the:
- suffering
- cruelty
- exploitation

of <u>All</u> forms of animals.

Vegans aim to do their part to end the suffering, cruelty and exploitation in all forms of animal use. This includes not participating or promoting any events or situations where another being will suffer or be exploited. The easiest way for us to show compassion as consumers is by putting our money towards the products and companies that we want to support and whose practices we agree with. By not spending our money on unethical goods or services we show that we do nor support these companies.

i ♥ my animal friends

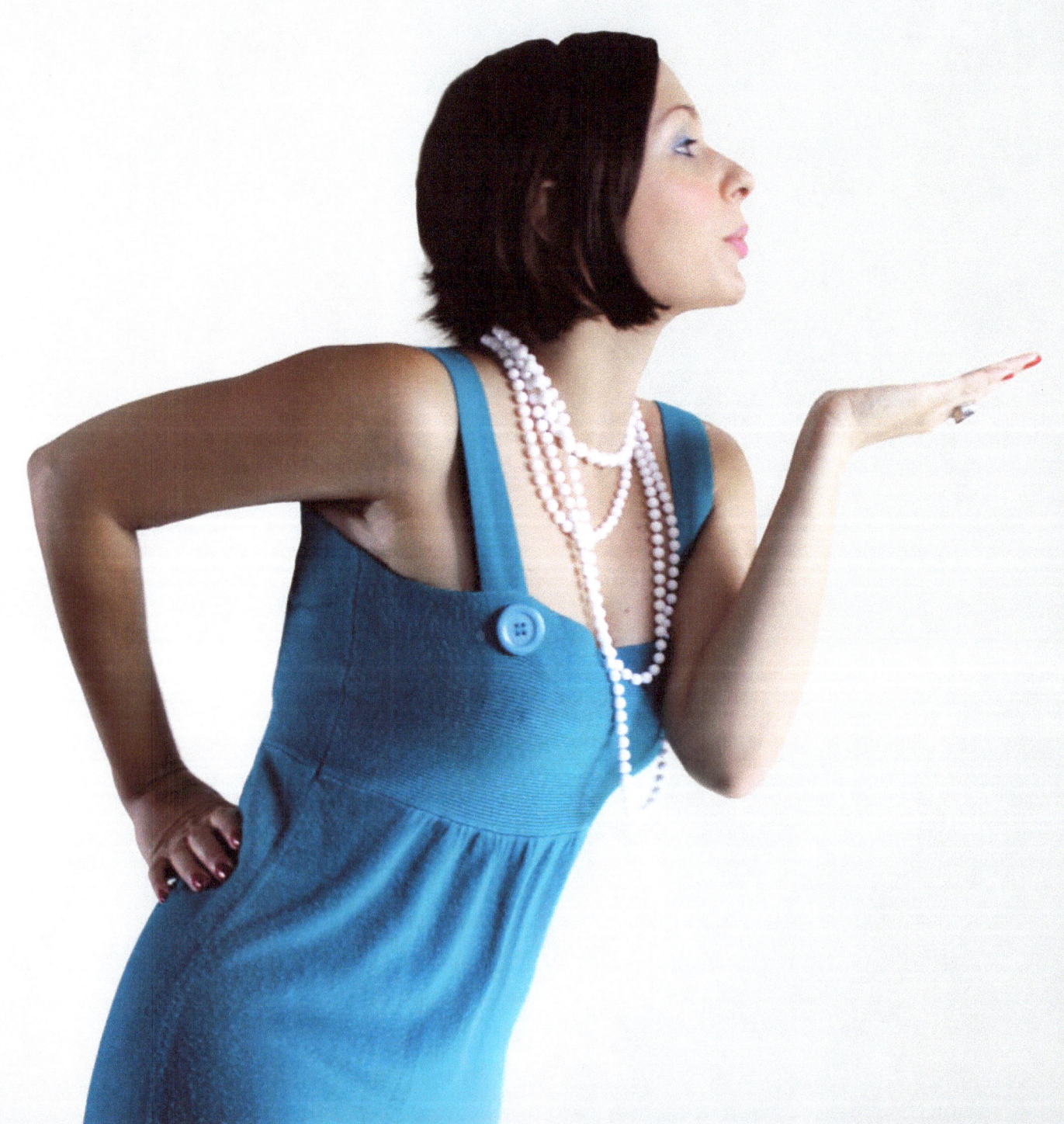

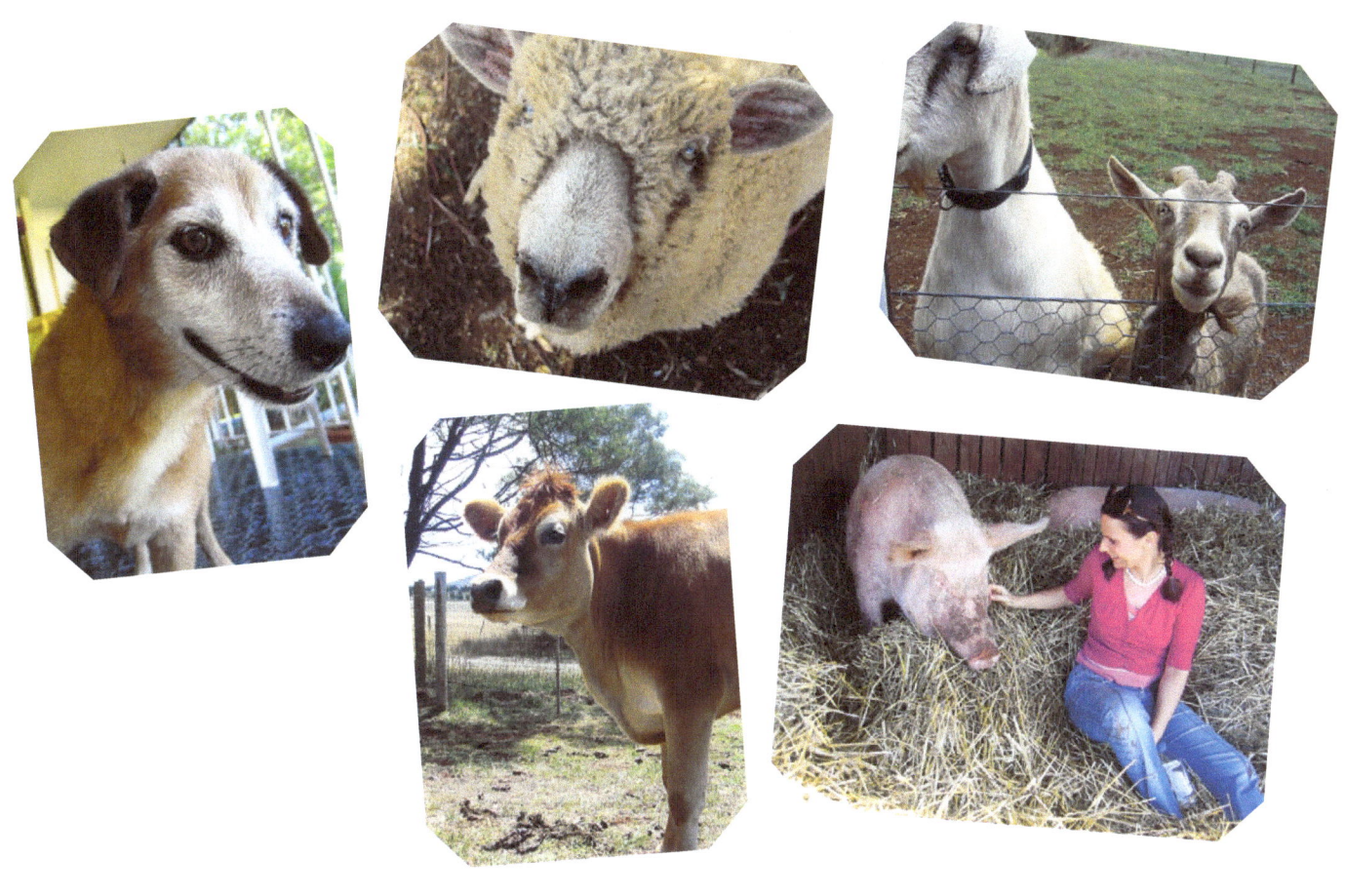

We should not kill, abuse or harm <u>ANY</u> beings on earth.

Reasons to be a VEGAN:

- animal rights and welfare concerns
- environmental and sustainable living
- ethical and moral reasons
- health issues
- spiritual and/or religious beliefs
- weight loss or control

There are many reasons why people decide to become a Vegan. They include:

- Animal rights and Welfare concerns
- Environmental and sustainable living
- Ethical and moral reasons
- Health issues
- Spiritual and/or Religious beliefs
- Weight loss or control

I became a vegan because I love my animal friends and I believe it's morally and ethically the right thing to do. I don't believe that we should kill, abuse or harm any beings on this earth, as we are here to take care of this world and all of the beings on it, and this includes each other.

What do vegans eat?

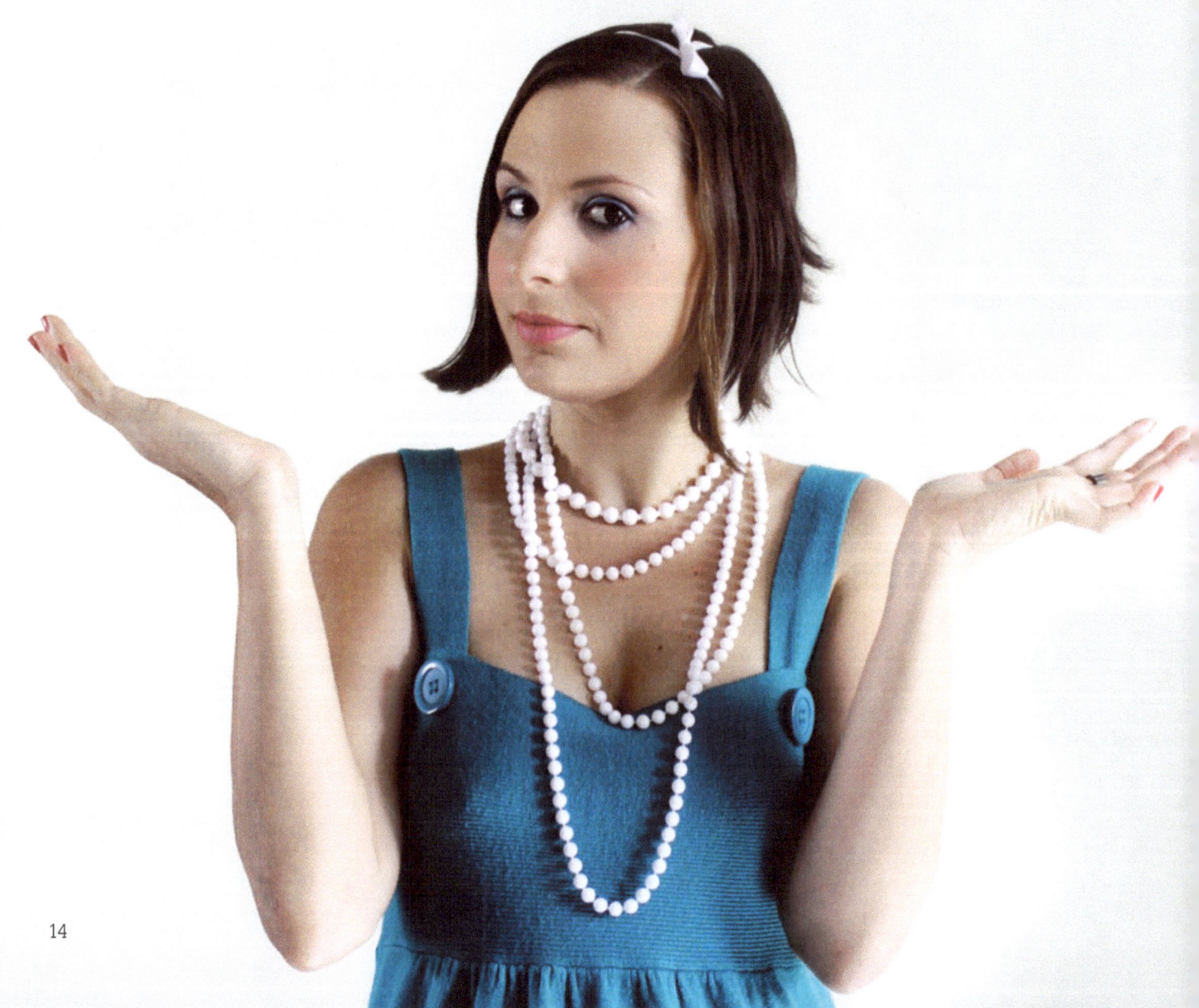

So many people ask me "What do Vegans eat?" so I'm going to show you!

The Basic foods staples for the vegan diet are:

- Fruit & Vegetables
- Whole grains
- Legumes & Pulses
- Nuts & Seeds

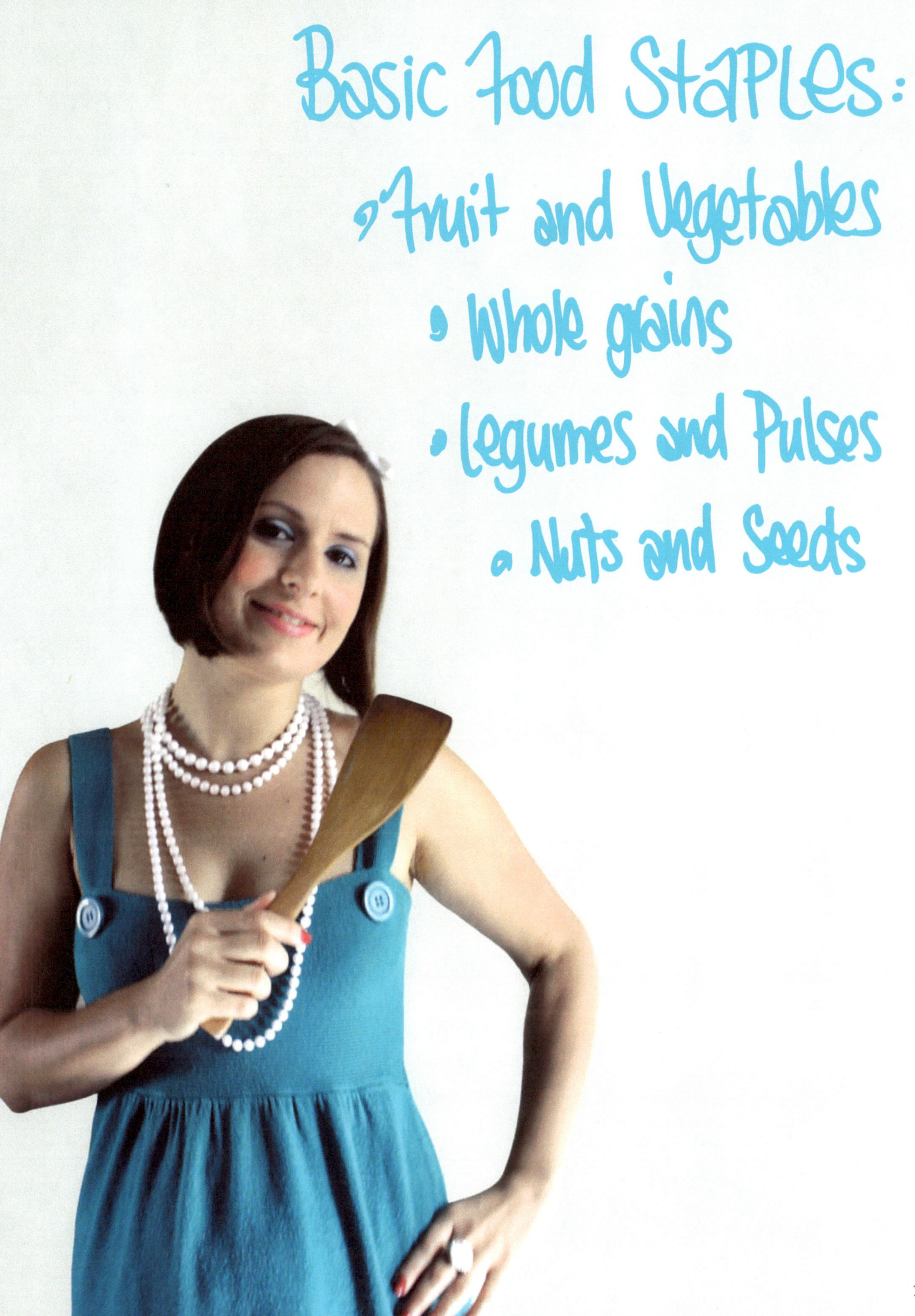

Fruit & Vegetables are a great source of fibre, essential vitamins and minerals and are critical to promoting good health. Make sure you eat all of the colours of the rainbow to ensure variety and the wide range of nutrients necessary for your body including folate, potassium, Vitamins A & C.

Fruit & Vegetables
- great source of fibre
- choose all the colours

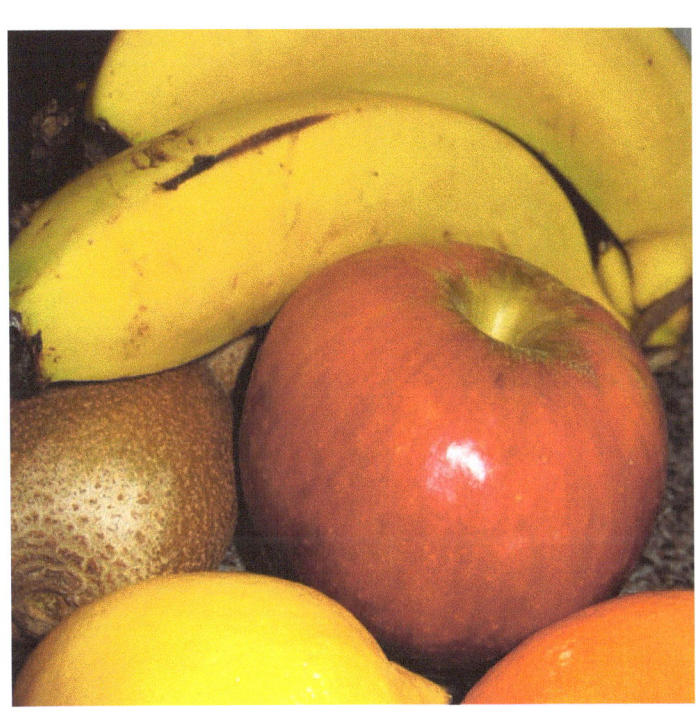
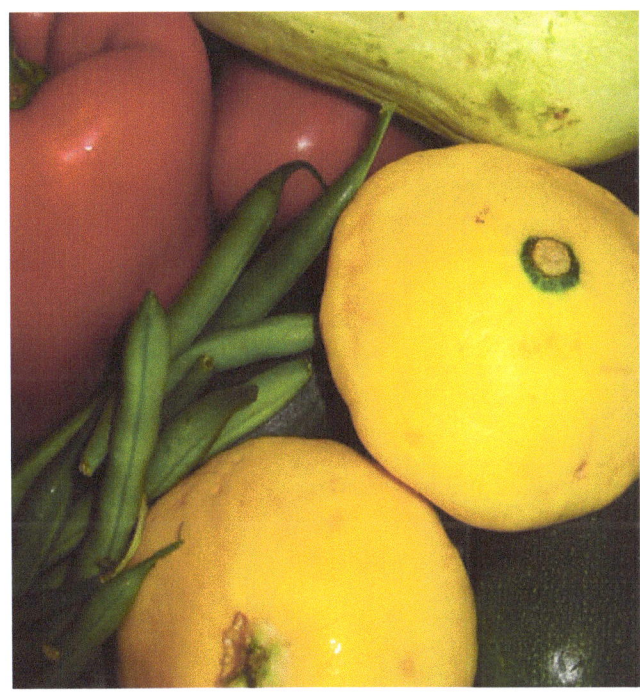

Dark green leafy vegetables are a great concentrated source of nutrition and contain many of our essential vitamins and minerals including Vitamins A, C, E, K, folate, iron, calcium, potassium and magnesium. Generally the darker the leaves the more nutrient dense. Examples include bok choy, chicory, dandelion greens, kale, spinach etc.

dark green leafy vegetables
eg. bok choy, Asian greens

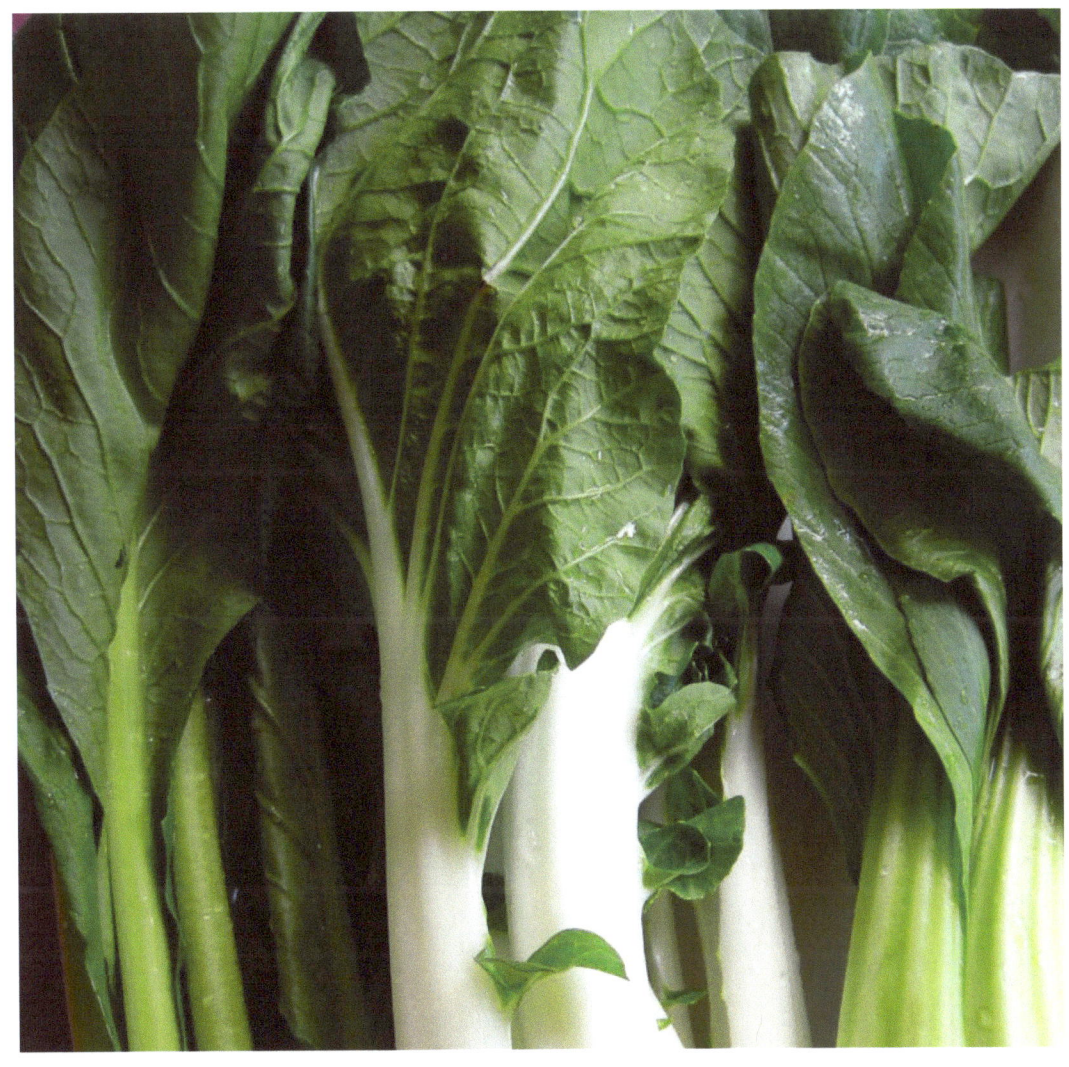

Whole grains are a great source of fibre and protein. Unlike refined and white products, whole grains have all their nutrients still intact. Whole grains are a low-glycaemic index (GI) food, which means that they are metabolised slower and don't cause extreme changes in blood sugar levels. This limits the highs and lows that contribute to snacking and sugar cravings. All grains should be rinsed before cooking and if possible soaked overnight to encourage ease of digestion. Examples of whole grains include: brown rice, wild rice, polenta, oats, quinoa, barley, rye, millet and more. Most grains should be cooked with the ratio of 1 cup of the grain to 2 cups of water.

WHOLE GRAINS

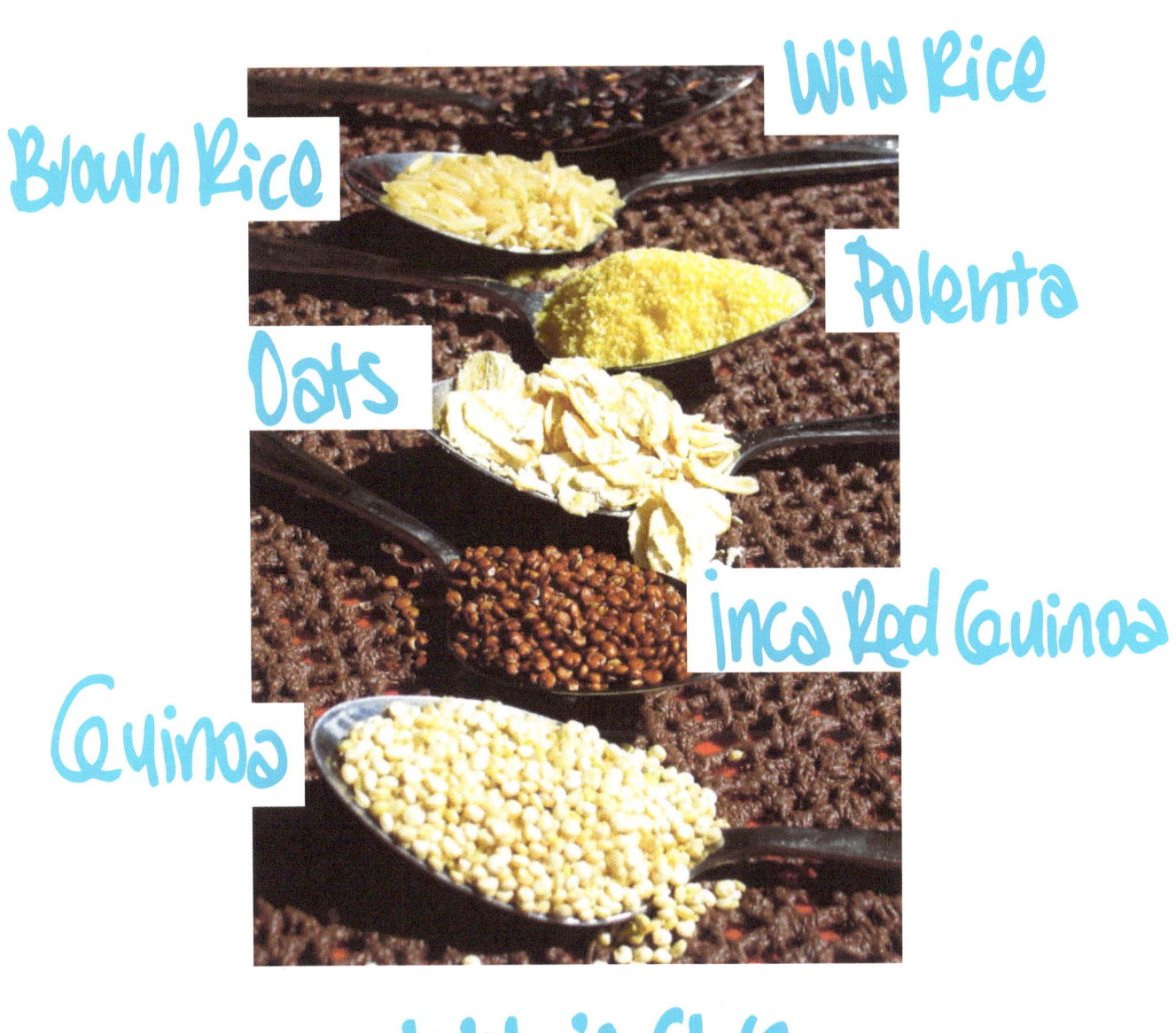

Brown Rice, Wild Rice, Polenta, Oats, Inca Red Quinoa, Quinoa

- high in fibre

Legumes & Pulses are high in fibre, carbohydrates, protein, and are a great addition to any diet. Most beans need to be washed thoroughly, soaked overnight and then cooked. Soak beans in at least three times their volume of water overnight. In the morning rinse and change the water a couple of times as this will get rid of the indigestible complex sugars that create gas in your intestine, and it also helps to cook the beans thoroughly.

Cover the beans with twice their volume of water and bring to the boil, reduce heat and simmer until soft. Cooking times vary, see the cooking tables on my website vivalavegan.net for more information. You can cook large batches of your favourite legumes and pulses and freeze them to use for cooking later on.

Legumes and Pulses

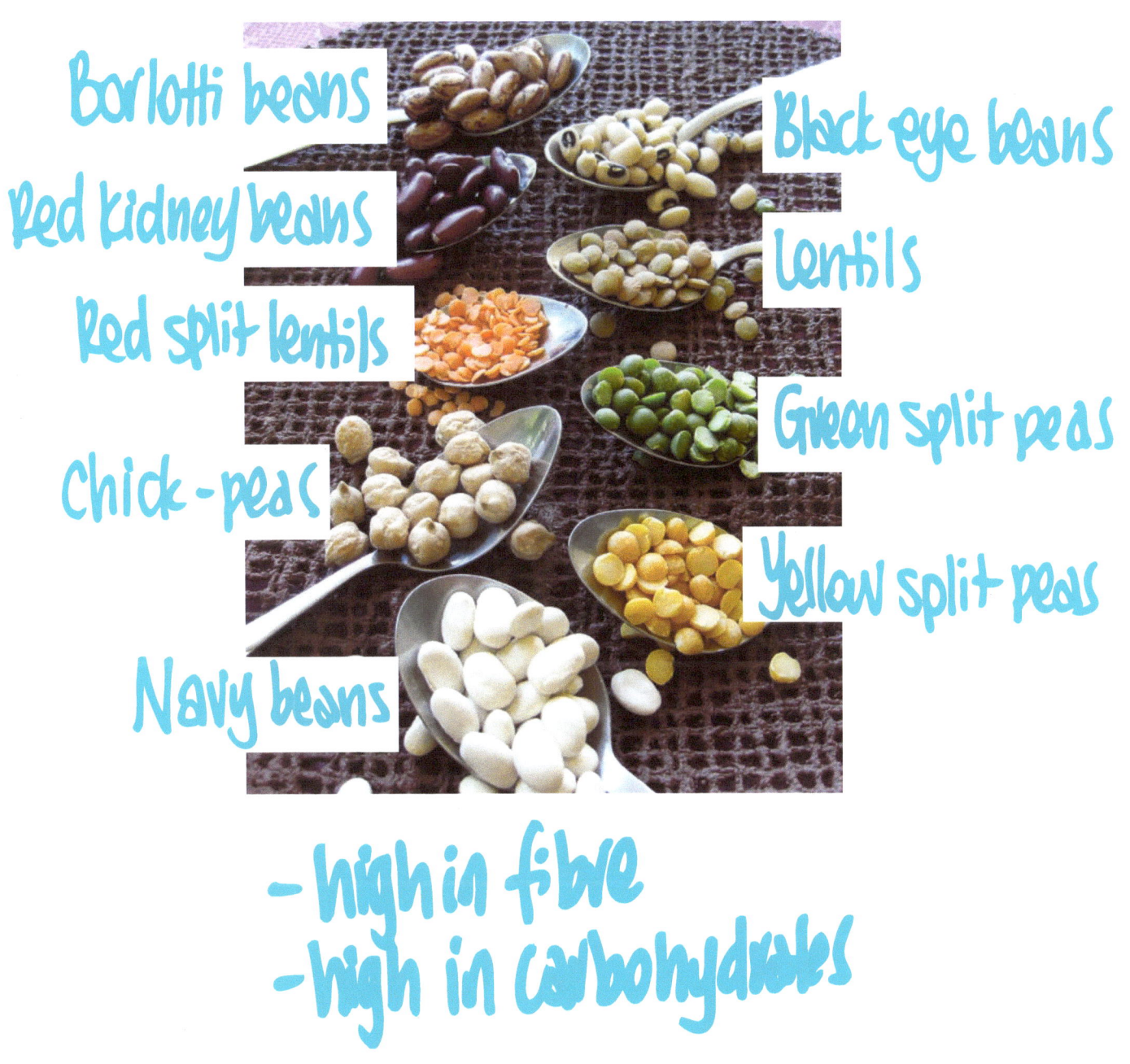

- Borlotti beans
- Red kidney beans
- Red split lentils
- Chick-peas
- Navy beans
- Black eye beans
- Lentils
- Green split peas
- Yellow split peas

- high in fibre
- high in carbohydrates

Nuts & Seeds are a quick and easy great source of protein, vitamins and nutrients. Different types include macadamia nuts, cashews, walnuts, linseeds, sesame seeds, pepitas (pumpkin seeds), Brazil nuts, almonds, pine nuts, hazelnuts, pecans, flax seeds, pistachos, sunflower seeds and more.

Keep in mind that some people are allergic to nuts, if so you will have to ensure that you get your protein, vitamins and minerals from the pulses and legumes, fruit and vegetables and whole grains that you consume. If you are overweight or watching your weight it's best not to eat nuts daily. Nuts are best kept in the fridge so they don't go rancid.

Nuts and Seeds

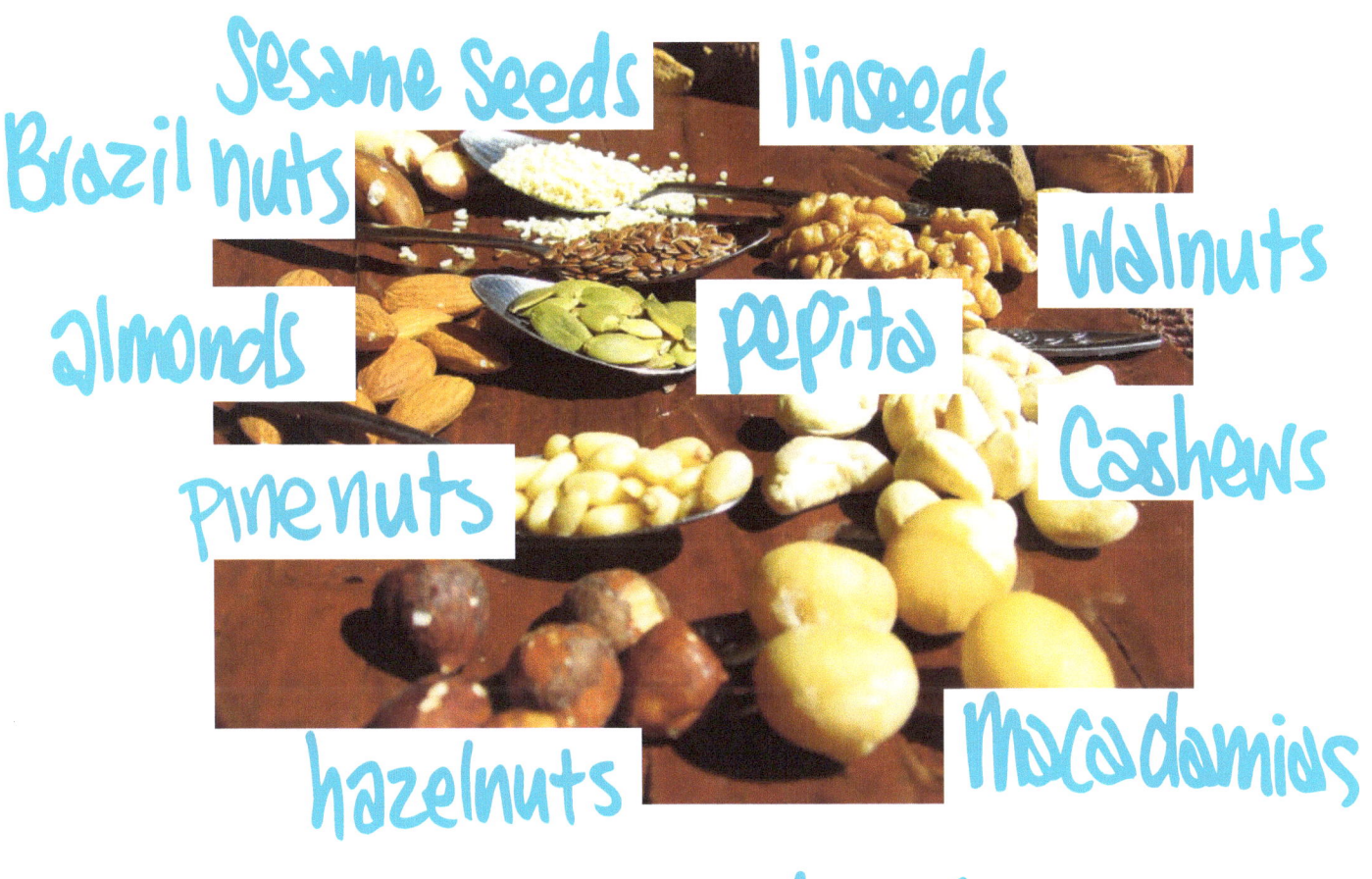

Sesame seeds, linseeds, Brazil nuts, walnuts, almonds, pepita, pine nuts, cashews, hazelnuts, macadamias

- quick and easy
- protein source

Vegan (whole) food is environmentally sustainable, ethical, delicious, nutritious and most of all, vegan food is cruelty-free!

Vegan food is:

- ethical
- delicious
- nutritious
- cruelty-free
- environmentally friendly

instead of Dairy milk
- soy milk
- oat milk
- brown rice milk
- almond & other nut milk

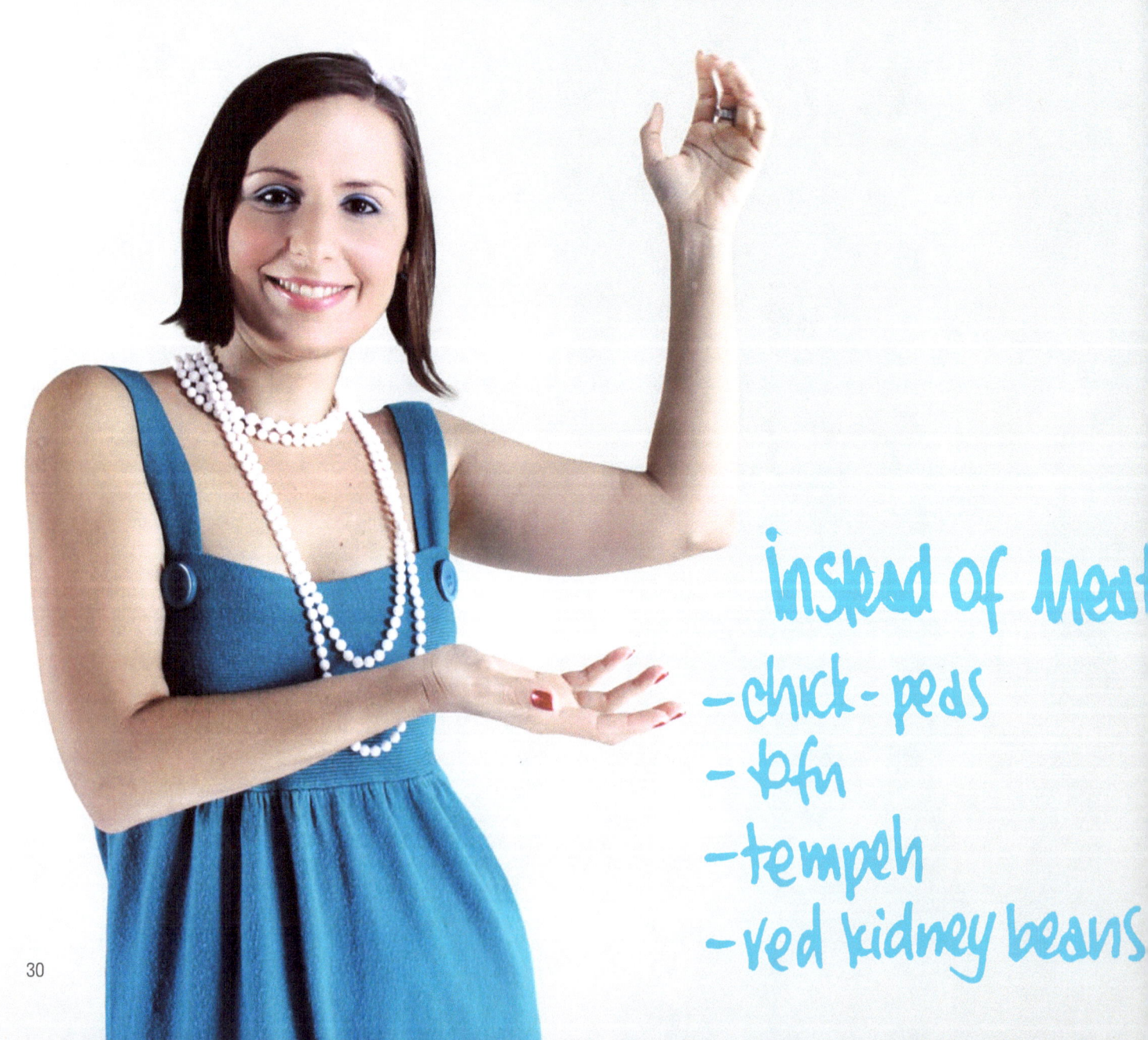

instead of Meat
- chick-peas
- tofu
- tempeh
- red kidney beans

There are many alternatives to the regular mainstream fare nowadays than what was available when I became vegan over 15 years ago. For example, instead of eating meat, choose to eat chickpeas, tofu, tempeh, red kidney beans and more. Instead of drinking dairy milk, choose soy milk, oat milk, brown rice milk, hemp milk, almond and other nut milks.

I run an interactive and informative website, vivalavegan.net with many different recipes online. I'm going to share some of the recipe photographs with you to inspire you to create some new meals at home.

my website:

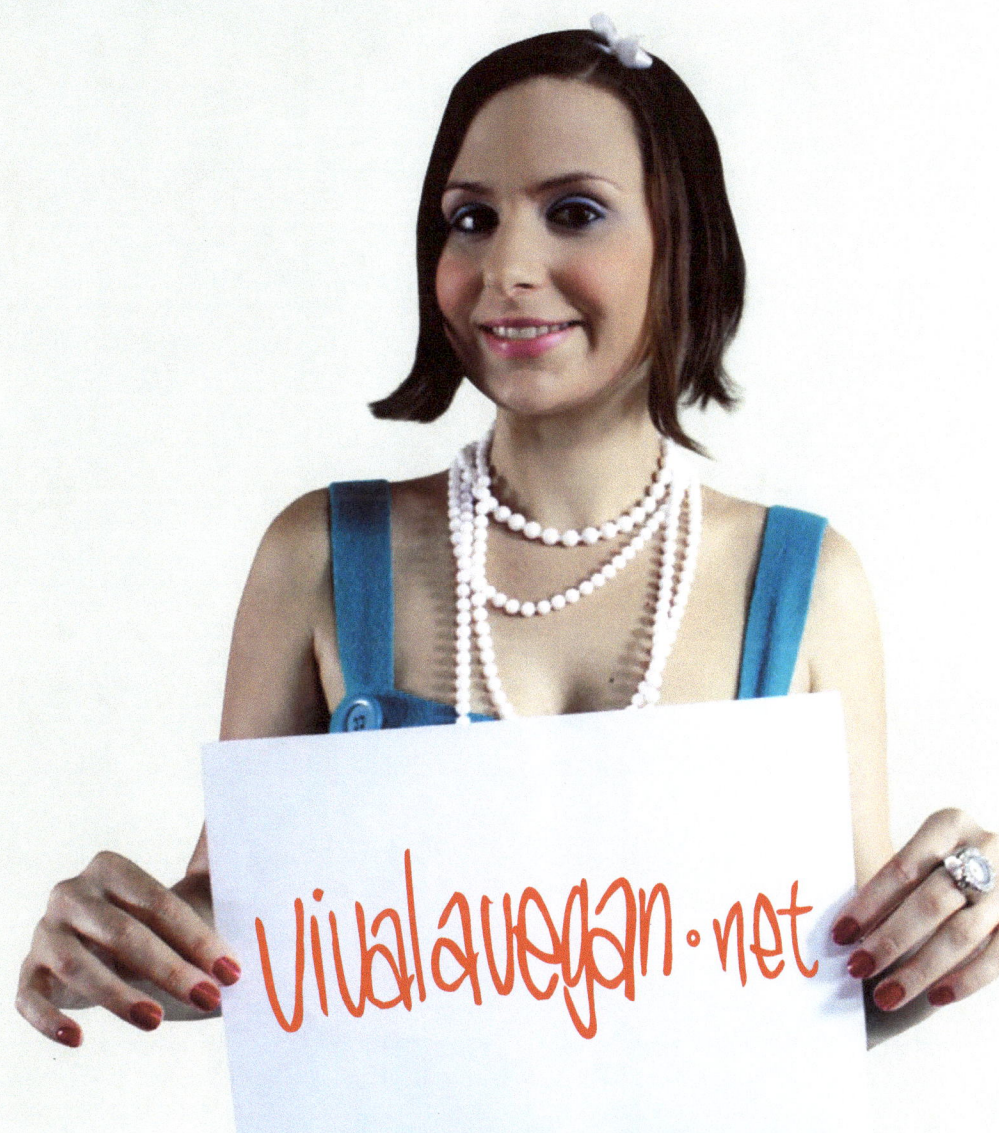

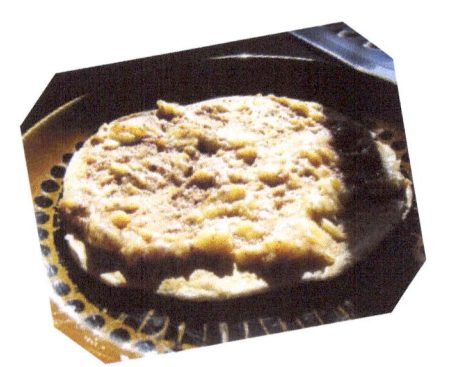 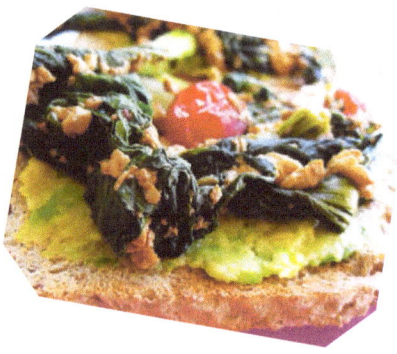 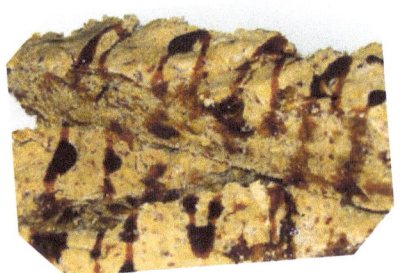

As breakfast is the most important meal of the day, it is necessary that you consume a nutritious breakfast that gives you the energy needed to start your day. Examples include buckwheat pancakes (savoury or banana and sweet), scrambled tofu, rye bread with molasses or with hummus, avocado and tomatoes.

Breakfast:

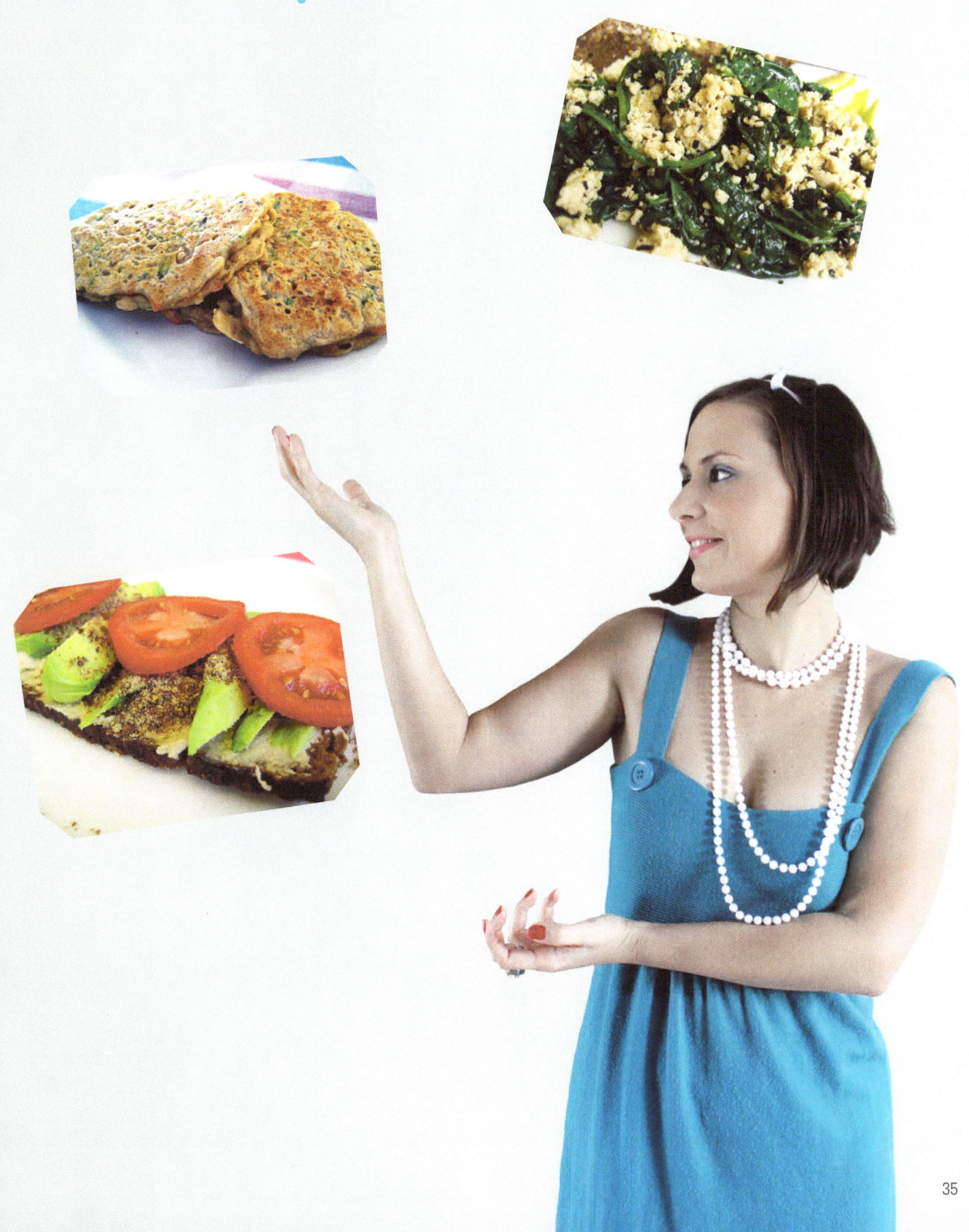

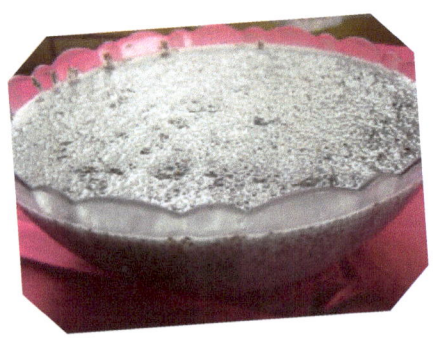

If you don't like a large meal for breakfast ensure you have some fruit or a vegetable juice. You can either eat a piece of fruit or make up a fruit salad. I always start the day with chia pudding and a fresh vegetable juice containing carrot, beetroot, ginger and cayenne pepper. There are so many different juices that you can create, so use your imagination!

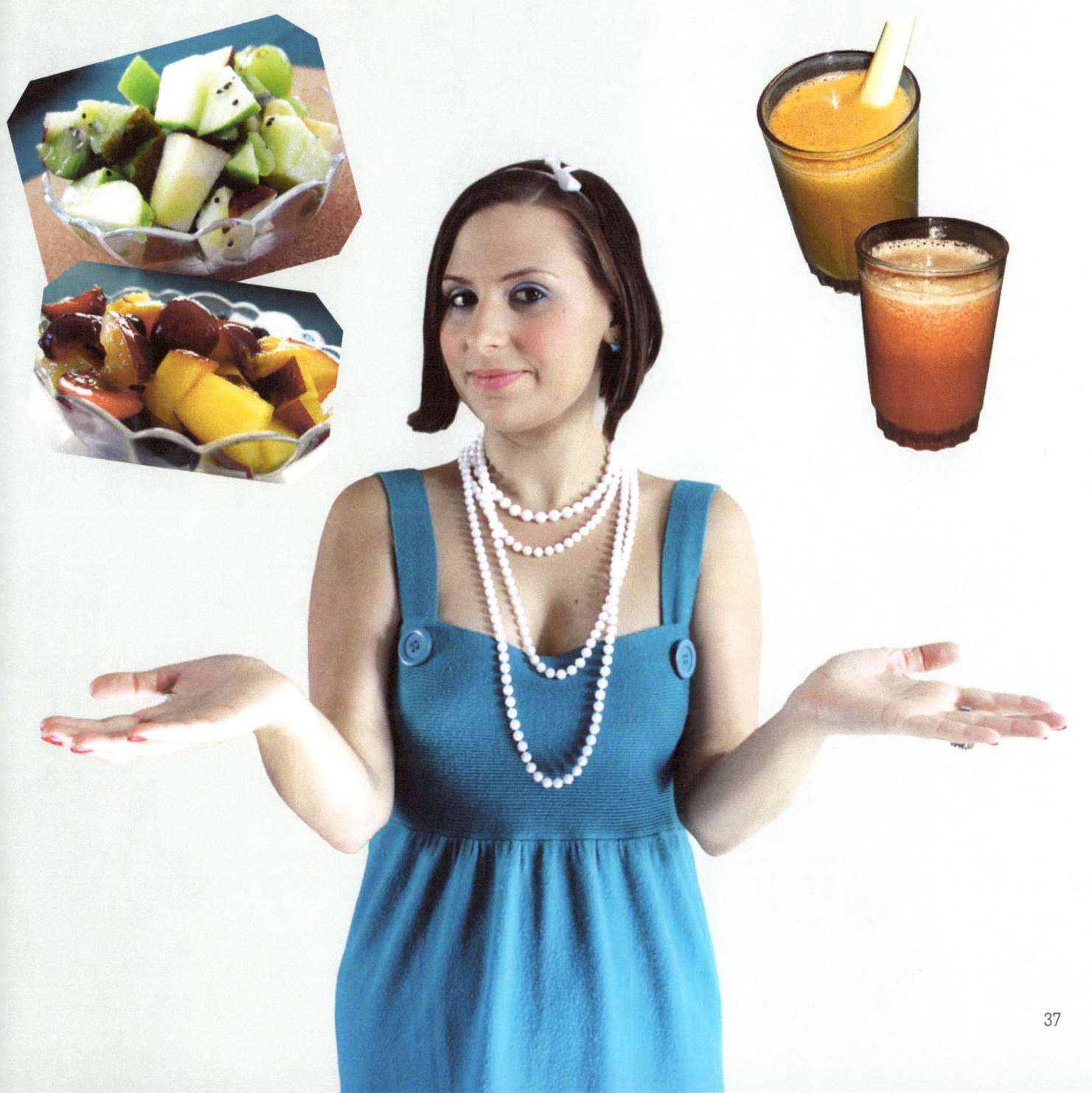

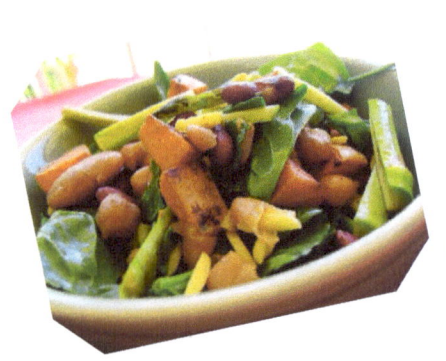 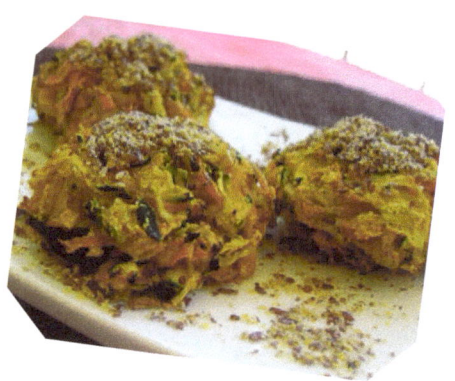 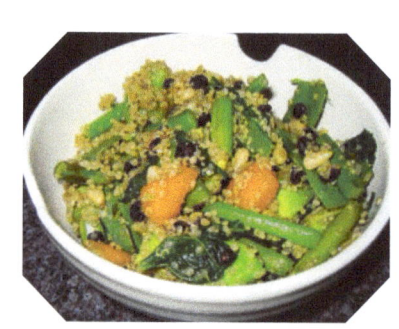

For lunch I generally like to have leftovers I've made from the night before. There are many options that you can have such as soup, stir-fries, currant and quinoa salad, dirty rice or vegetables with pumpkin and almond sauce.

Salads are quick and easy to prepare such as the sweet potato and mixed bean salad or vegetable and chickpea salad. Also tomatoes and herbs on rye bread or chickpea patties are great for lunch.

LUNCH:

Salads
Snacks

39

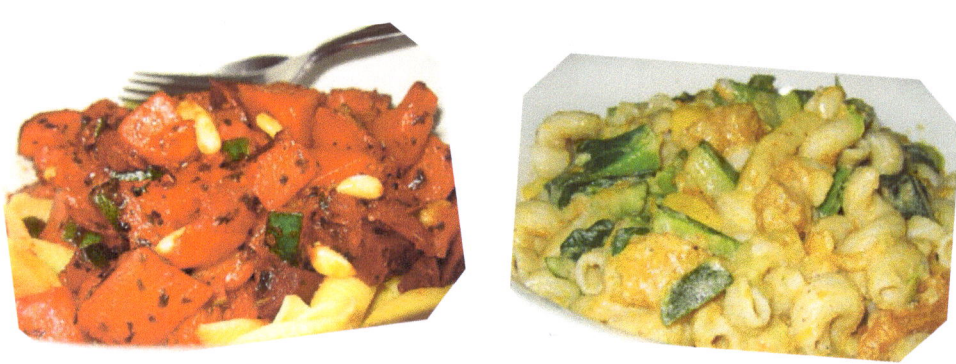

There are many different types of meals you can make for your dinner. Whatever your family's favourite meal is, I'm certain there is a more ethical vegan version. For example some pasta dishes including Beet pasta with pine nuts, lasagne, garlic gnocchi, veggie bake and more.

DINNER: PASTA

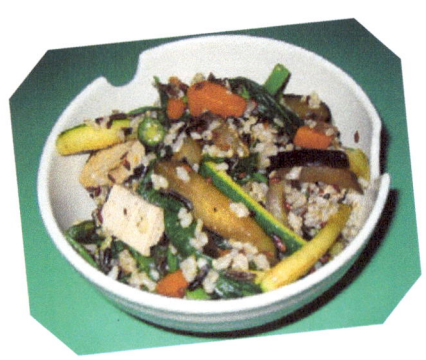 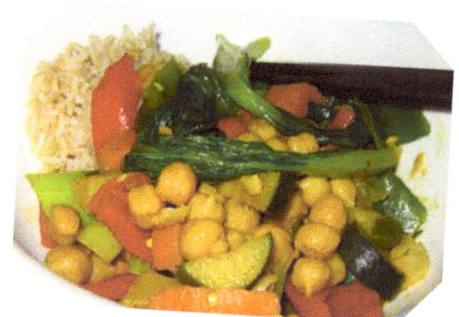

Some examples of rice dishes include Wild rice with Mediterranean vegetables, fried rice, stir fries, as well as various vegetable curries. You are only limited by your imagination.

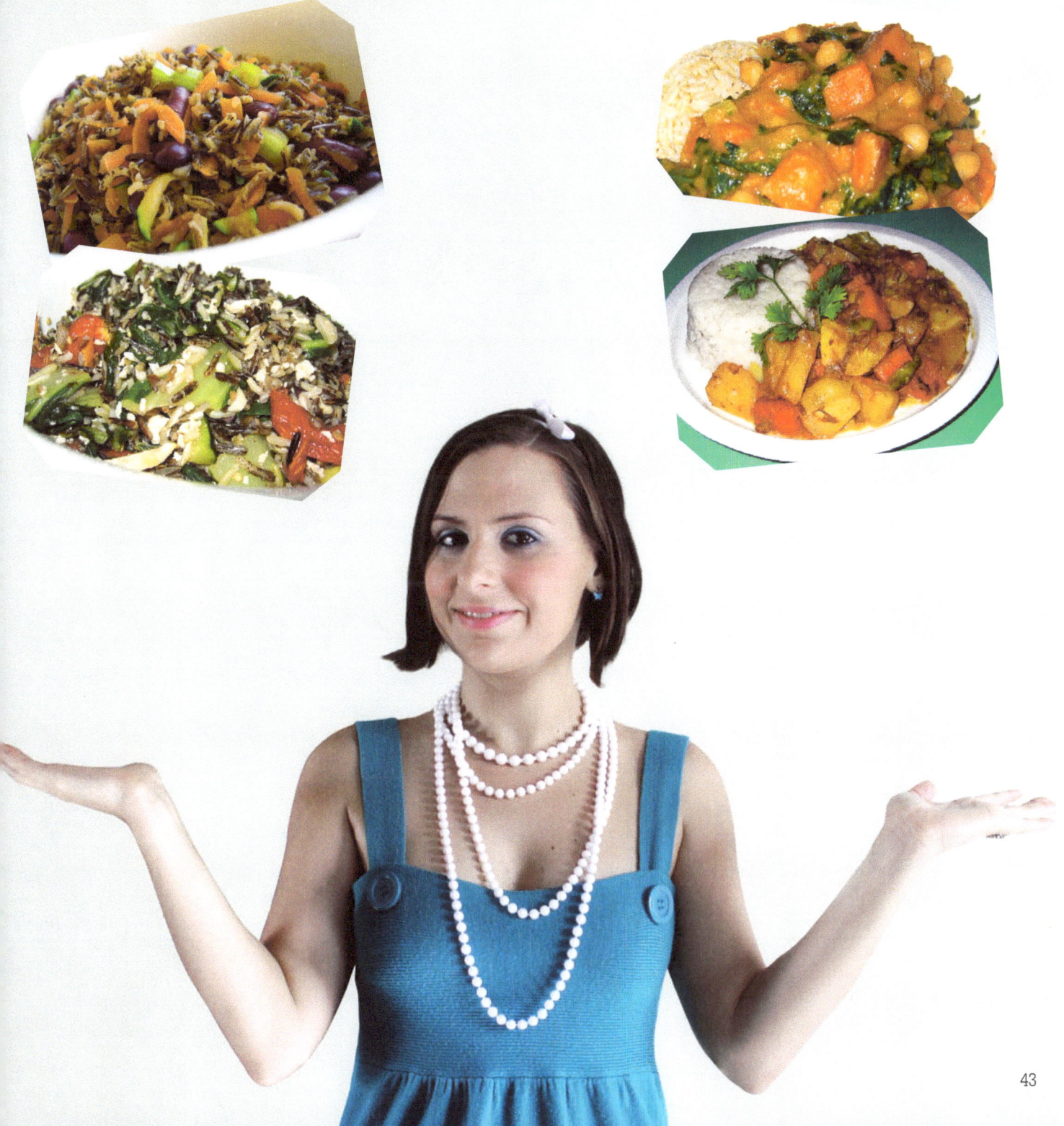

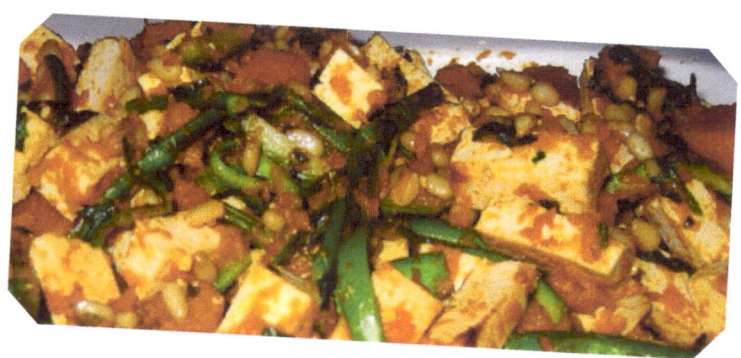

Stir-fries are so quick and easy to cook. Be creative with what you cook, use anything in your fridge or cupboard. Think of colourful, in season vegetables, plus don't forget the grains, legumes and/or nuts.

Stir-fries:

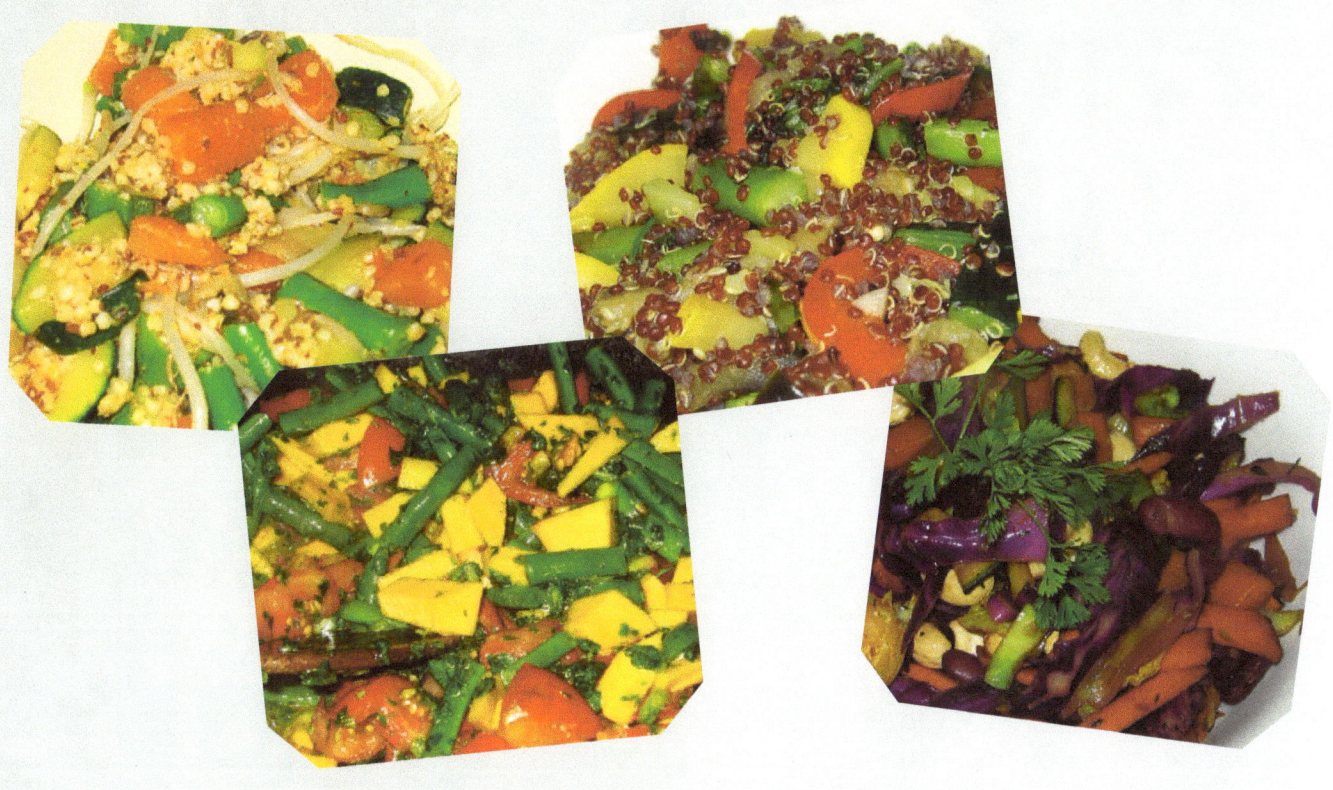

- easy
- quick to cook
- use anything
- be creative

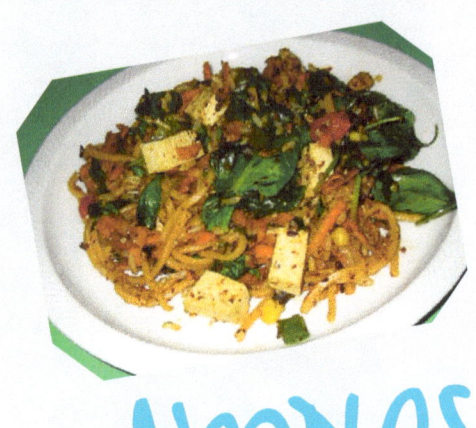
NOODLES

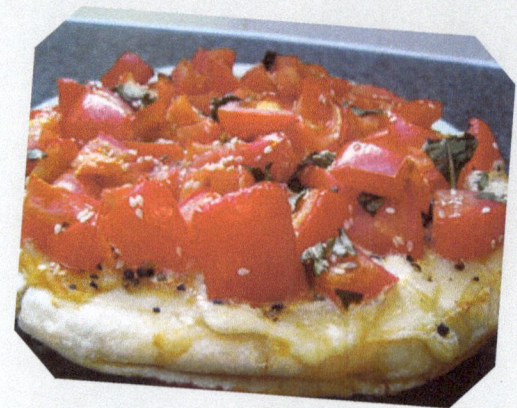
PIZZA

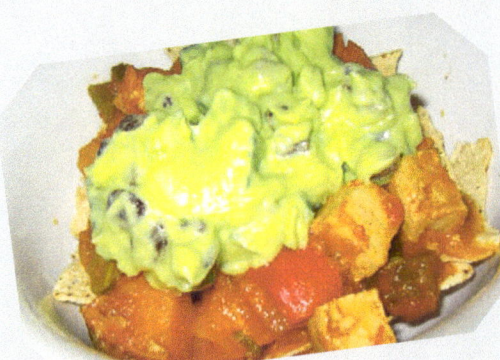
NACHOS

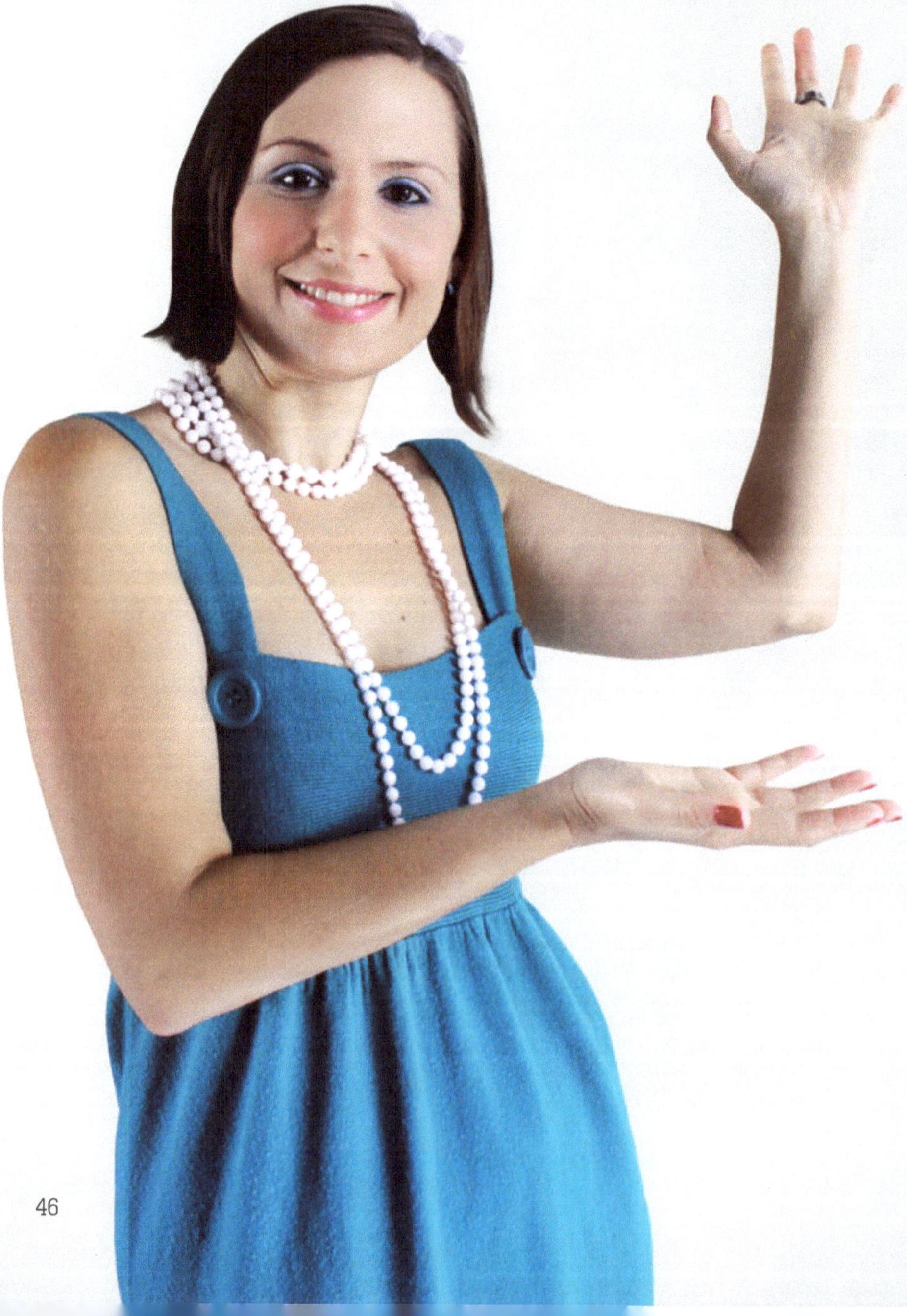

Other quick and easy to cook meals include noodle dishes, pizza and nachos. Be creative with your meals. You can covert anything into a vegan meal!

Other ideas include: curry puffs, savoury pancakes, kebabs, veggie stacks, polenta and date cakes with stir-fried veggies. You can get all the recipes I've featured here on my vivalavegan.net website, my detox diet e-book, my recycled recipe cards, plus keep your eyes open for some other book releases in the not-so-distant future.

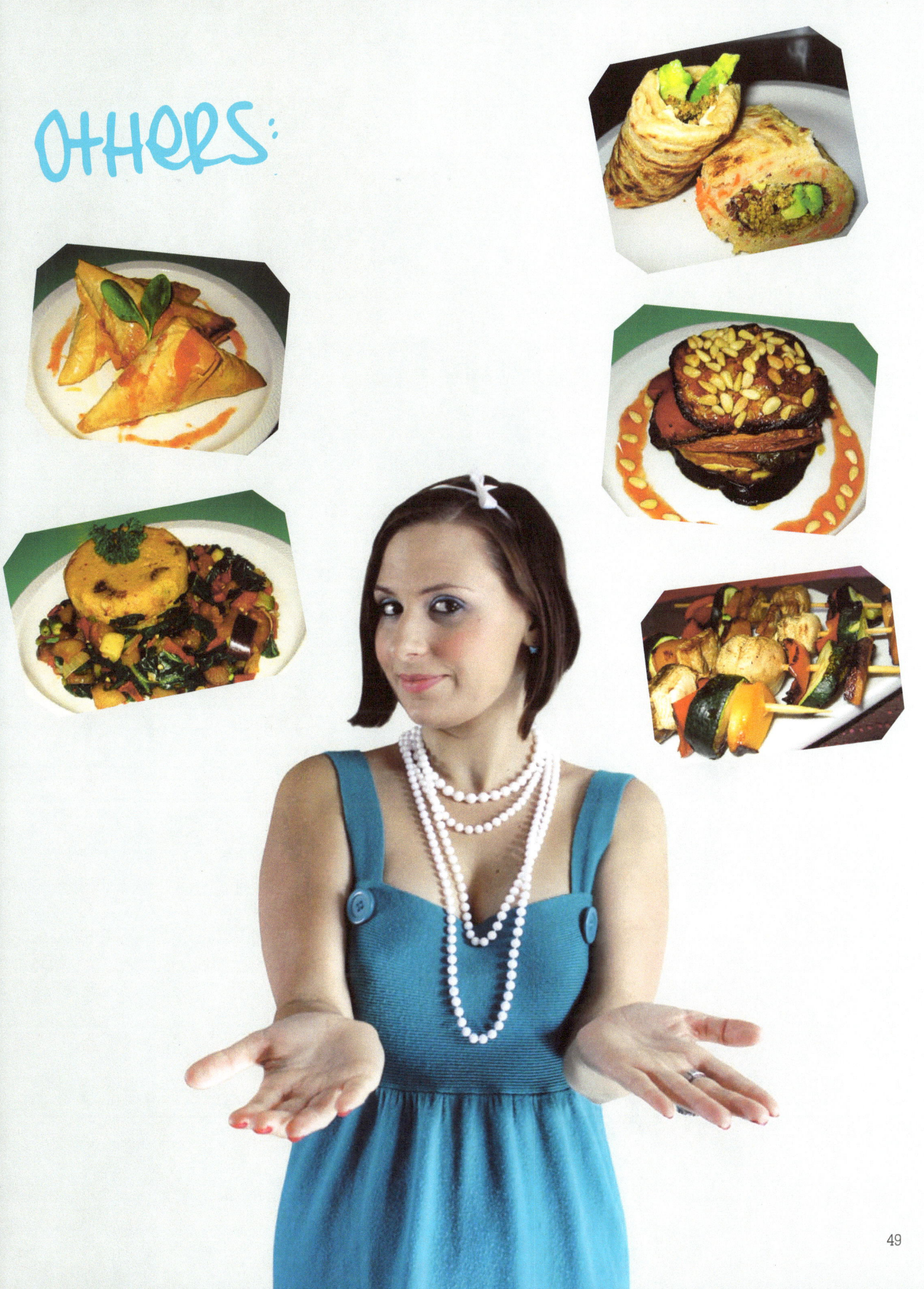

You **CAN** get all the vitamins, minerals and nutrients from a well-balanced, low fat, wide variety plant-based (vegan) diet.

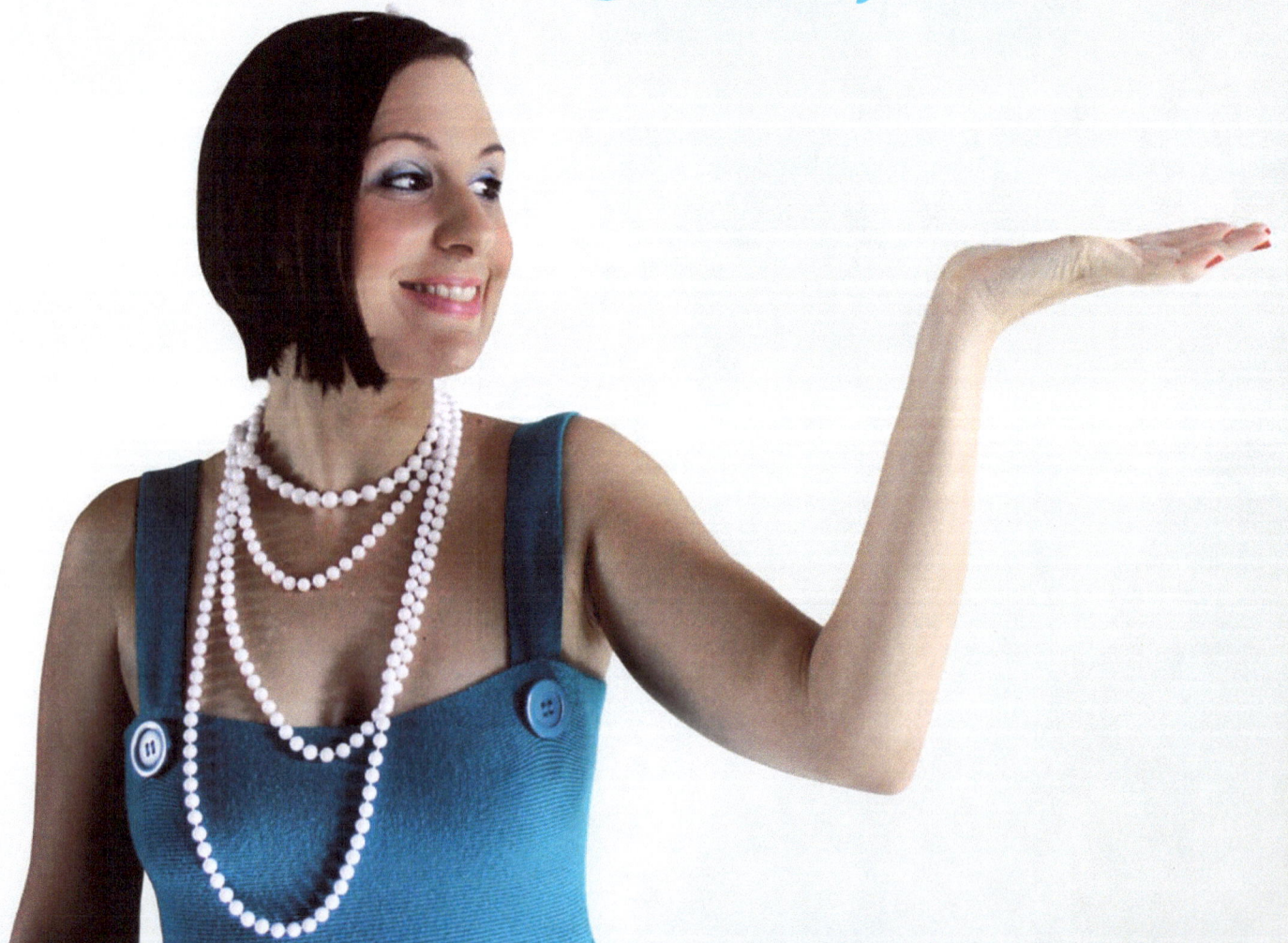

You can get all of the vitamins, minerals and nutrients you need from a well-balanced plant-based diet. If you were previously getting your nutrients from animal products, then you need to know where to get the same nutrients from plant-based foods. If you are unsure, make sure you do some research and educate yourself to the vegan sources of the nutrients you need.

The basic food staples of the vegan diet are whole grains, pulses and legumes, nuts and seeds as well as fruit and vegetables. These provide all of the vitamins and minerals that we need. Vitamin B12 is also needed and a bit controversial, as some people believe you should be able to get B12 from a well-balanced, varied plant-based diet. There are others who are well-reputed and believe the only way to accurately get vitamin B12 is to supplement.

If you have been a vegan for over five years, have digestive or malabsorption problems, are worried or even just curious about vitamin B12 I would suggest you get your doctor to do a saliva or blood test to check your levels. Ensure you consume products fortified with vitamin B12 and/or use a B12 supplement. I have some more information on this controversial vitamin on vivalavegan.net

Minerals:
Calcium, Iodine, Iron, Magnesium, Potassium, Selenium Silicon, Zinc

Vitamins:
A
B
C
D
E
K

Vitamin B12
fortified products

You can get all of your protein needs if you are eating a well-balanced, varied, plant-based diet and consuming all of the vegan staples. Protein provides the body with energy and is essential for growth and development. When the body makes protein, it needs a variety of amino acids, the building blocks of protein, for this process. Complete proteins contain all the 8 essential amino acids for example quinoa, chickpeas, green leafy vegetables, lentils, millet, nuts, pumpkin and sesame seeds and tahini, soy products and more.

Carbohydrates are the fuel of life and provide our bodies the energy needed to function. Complex carbohydrates include fibre and starches, for example vegetables, whole grains, peas and beans. Complex carbohydrates are low-glycaemic index (GI) foods. These low GI foods metabolise slower and don't cause extreme changes in blood sugar levels like the simple carbohydrates. Fibre also lowers blood cholesterol and stabilises blood sugar levels.

Carbohydrates
- fuel of life
- provide energy
- complex carbs are low-Glycaemic index

Protein:

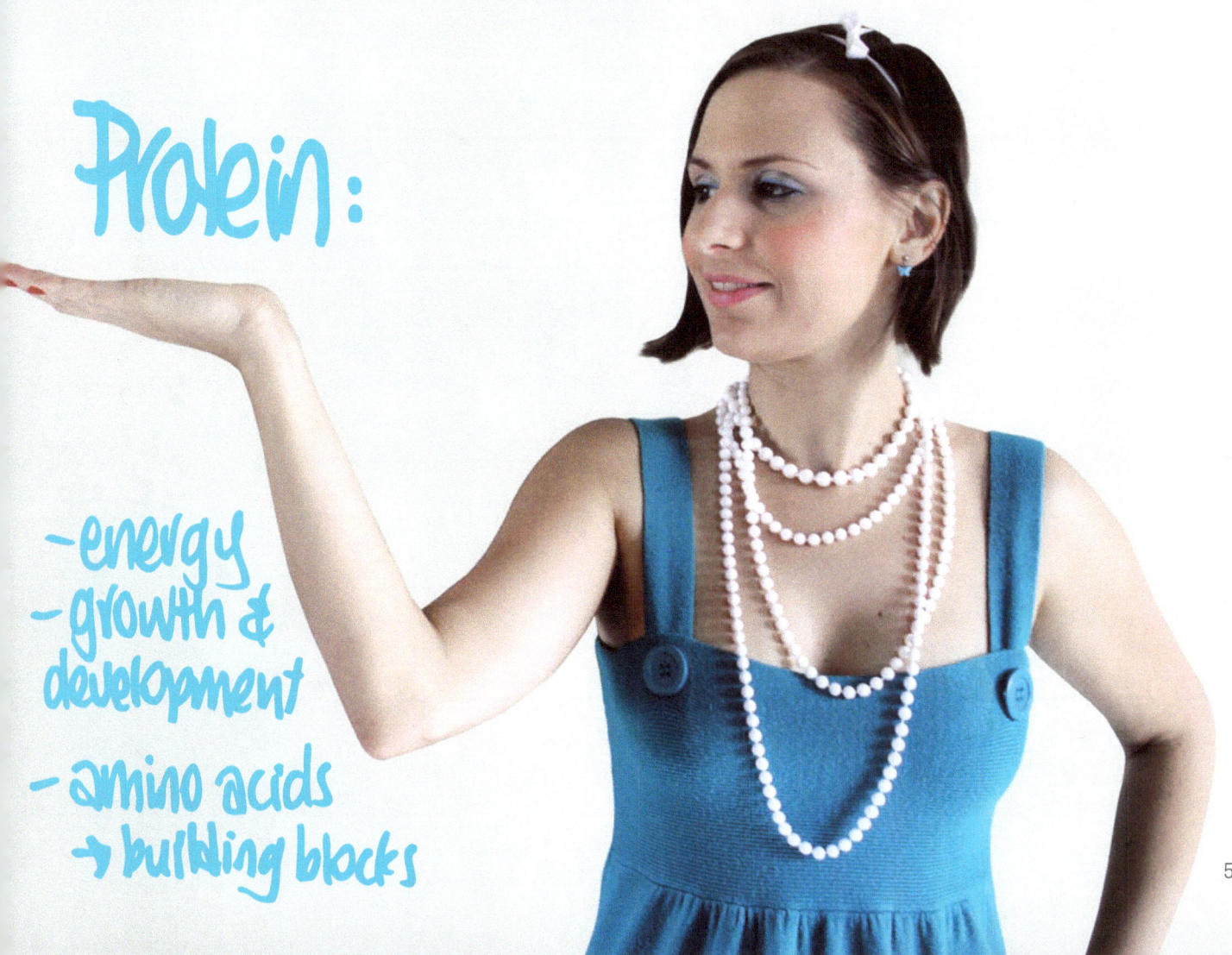

- energy
- growth & development
- amino acids → building blocks

Iron:
- haemoglobin production
- prevents anaemia

Water:
- 70% of bodies
- all functions in our bodies

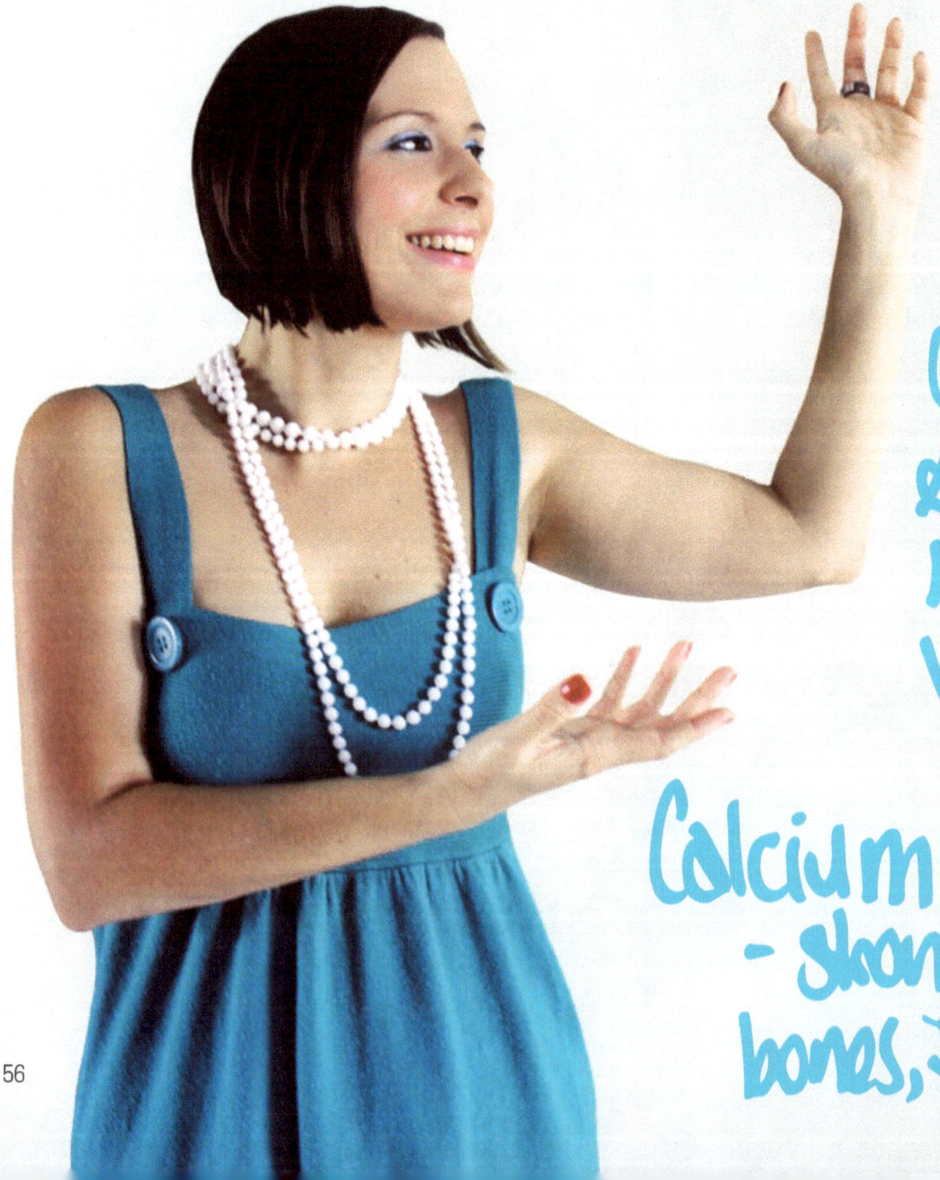

Essential Fatty Acids:
(Omega 3s & 6s)
avocado
Nuts and seeds
Vegetable oils

Calcium:
- strong & healthy bones, teeth & nails

Other important nutrients include Iron, which is needed for haemoglobin production, prevention of anaemia and proper metabolism of B vitamins. Sources include: dried fruit, whole grains, dark green leafy vegetables, nuts and seeds, legumes. Combine these sources with foods high in vitamin C to increase the absorption of iron.

Calcium is necessary for building strong and healthy bones, teeth and nails. Sources include: almonds, blackstrap molasses, brown rice, chick peas, figs, dark green leafy vegetables, lentils, millet, oats, quinoa, rye, seaweed, sesame seeds (tahini), soy beans, soy milk (especially if fortified), spinach and tofu.

As our bodies are made up of at least 70% water, it is very important to ensure that your body is well-hydrated. Water is involved in every function of the body, from transporting nutrients and waste products to maintaining proper body temperature. The water-soluble vitamins, B complex and C need water for their utilisation.

Certain types of fats are necessary for energy and supporting growth. There are three major categories of fatty acids: saturated, polyunsaturated and monounsaturated. Saturated fats are found mostly in animal products but also in coconut oil, palm kernel oil and vegetable shortening. Saturated fats raise blood cholesterol levels, so eat very little if any of these fats. Some polyunsaturated fats can be consumed such as corn, soybean, safflower and sunflower oils. Stick to monounsaturated vegetable and nut oils such as olive, peanut or sunflower oil.

I ♡ Quinoa

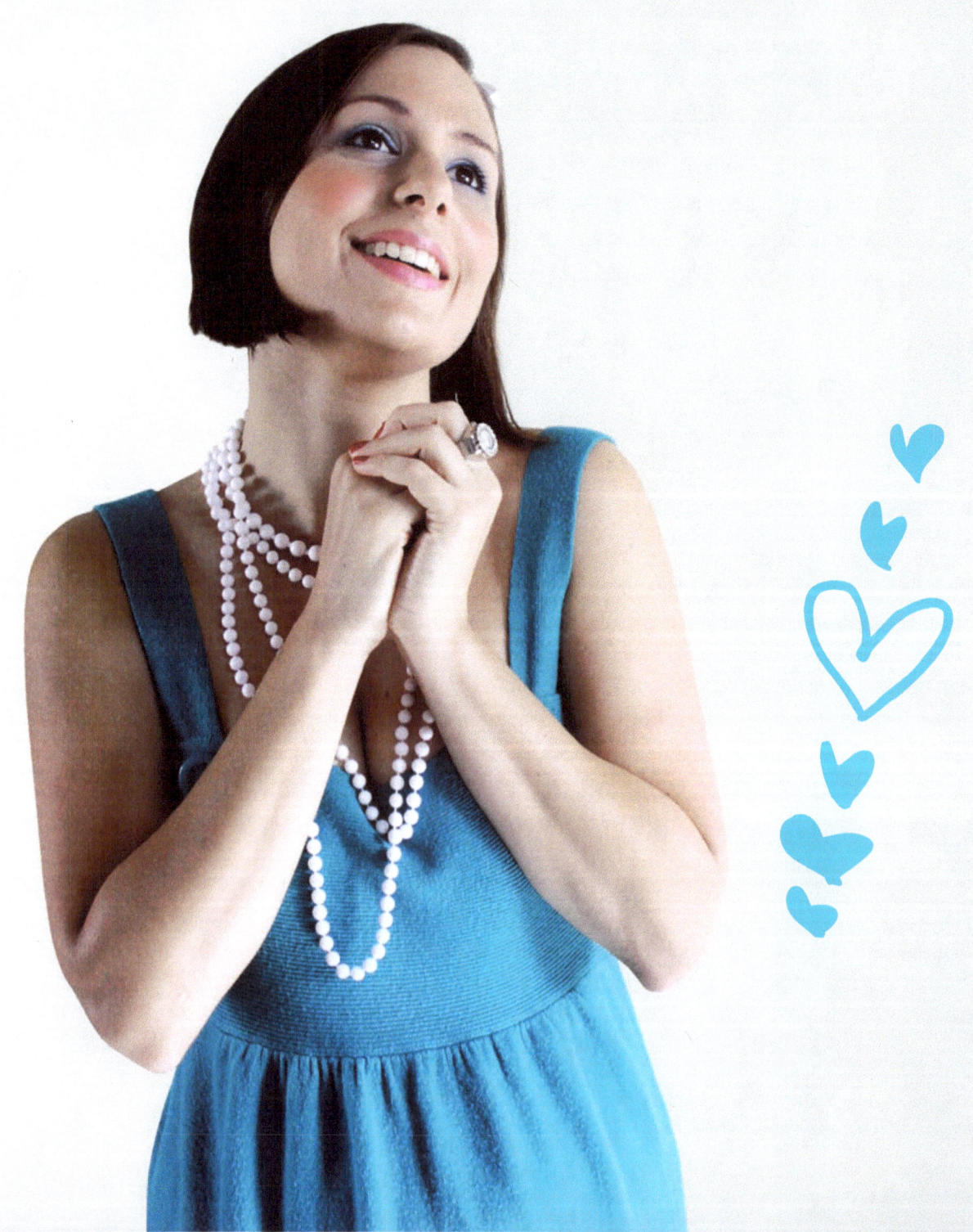

I am not ashamed in the slightest to confess my love of this amazing and ever so versatile alternative seed - not really a grain - my favourite quinoa. Years ago when I first discovered this ancient Inca grain, not many people had heard of the name let alone knew how to pronounce it (keen-wa.) Nowadays a lot more people know of this great seed which can be used as you would a grain. I believe it will be one of those "new super foods" heavily marketed in mainstream media in the coming years. There are three different versions of quinoa to buy: white, red and black, as well as quinoa flour, flakes and pasta. When quinoa has been cooked, a white rim forms on the periphery of the grain and it just looks beautiful.

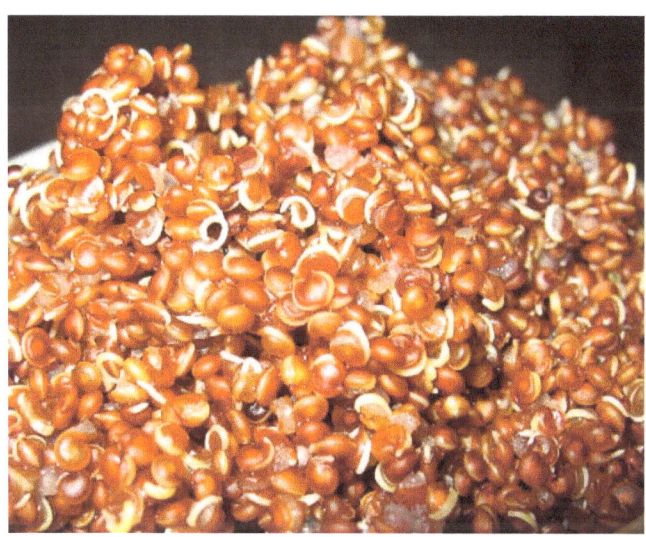

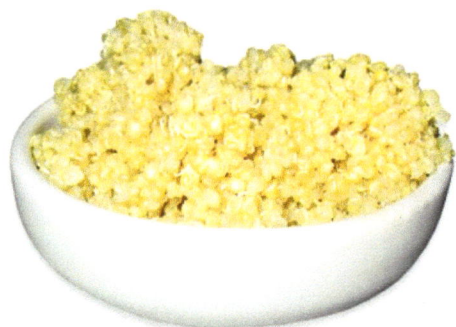

The quinoa seed comes from the Andes Mountains in South America and it was one of the staple foods of the Inca people. Quinoa is a complete protein meaning it contains all of the essential amino acids as well as having more protein than any other grain/seed. It can be used in any recipe where rice would normally be used. Quinoa is a very light ingredient that is easily digested and quick and easy to cook. Cook as you would any other grains: 1 cup of the grain to two cups of water. Another easy way to cook quinoa is by using a thermos: combine quinoa and boiling water and leave overnight. The mixture will be ready for the morning when you rise.

Quinoa:
- high levels of protein
- energy food
- easy to cook
- red and white
- great alternative grain

♥♥♥♡♥♥

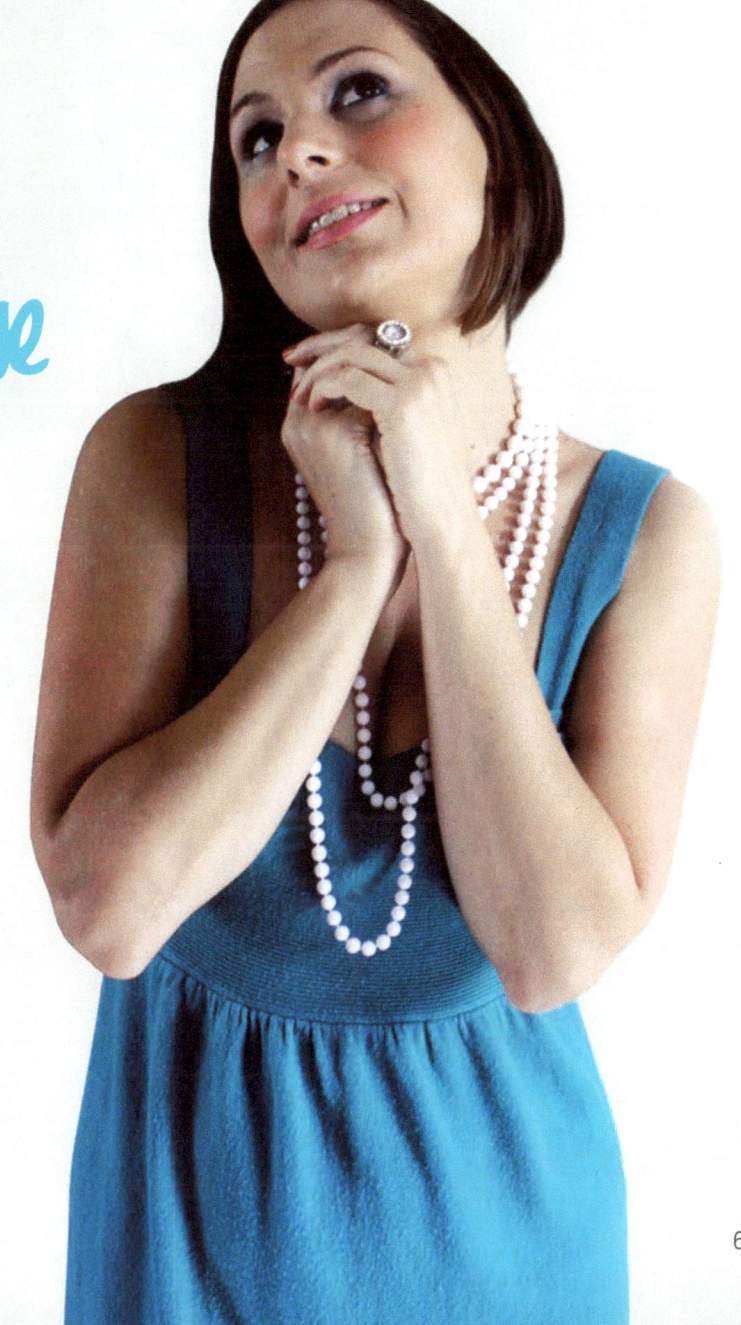

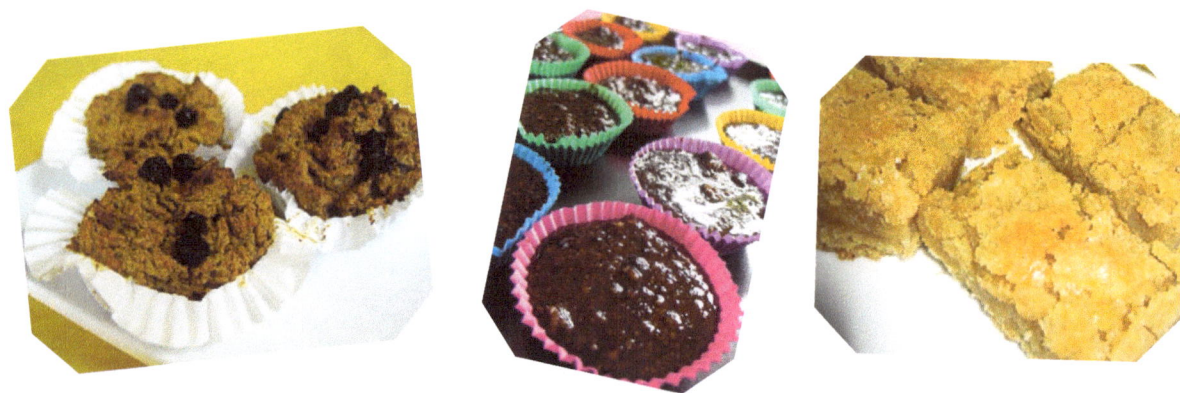

There is also a vast amount of vegan versions of desserts and sweets. Here I have my chocolate and seasonal fruit pie, walnut shortbread, the healthy carrot and currant muffins, chocolate shortbread and raw chocolate. If you have a favourite dessert, I'm sure there's a vegan version. Keep in mind to try and be as healthy as possible and eat as low fat as you can.

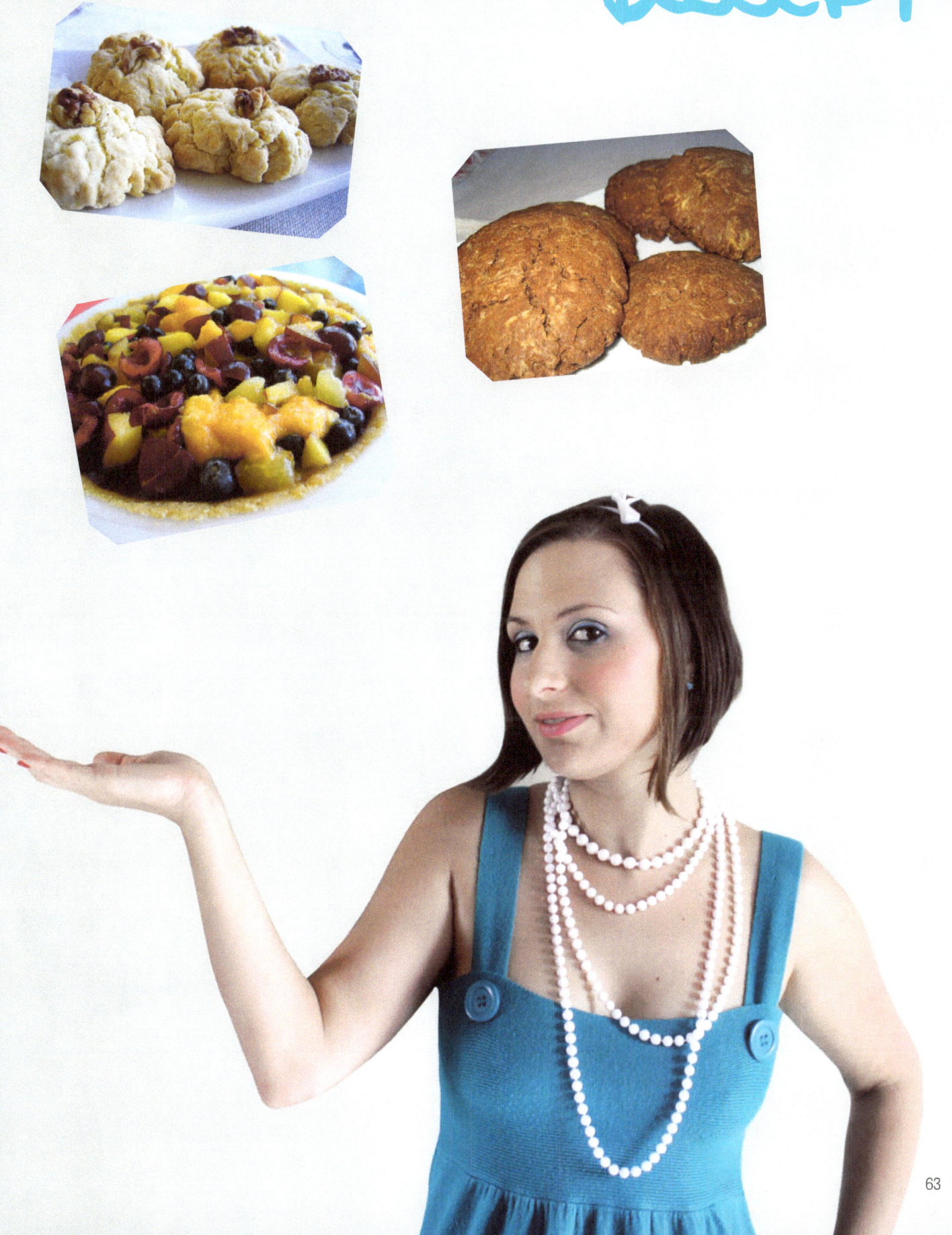

PLUS MORE DESSERTS

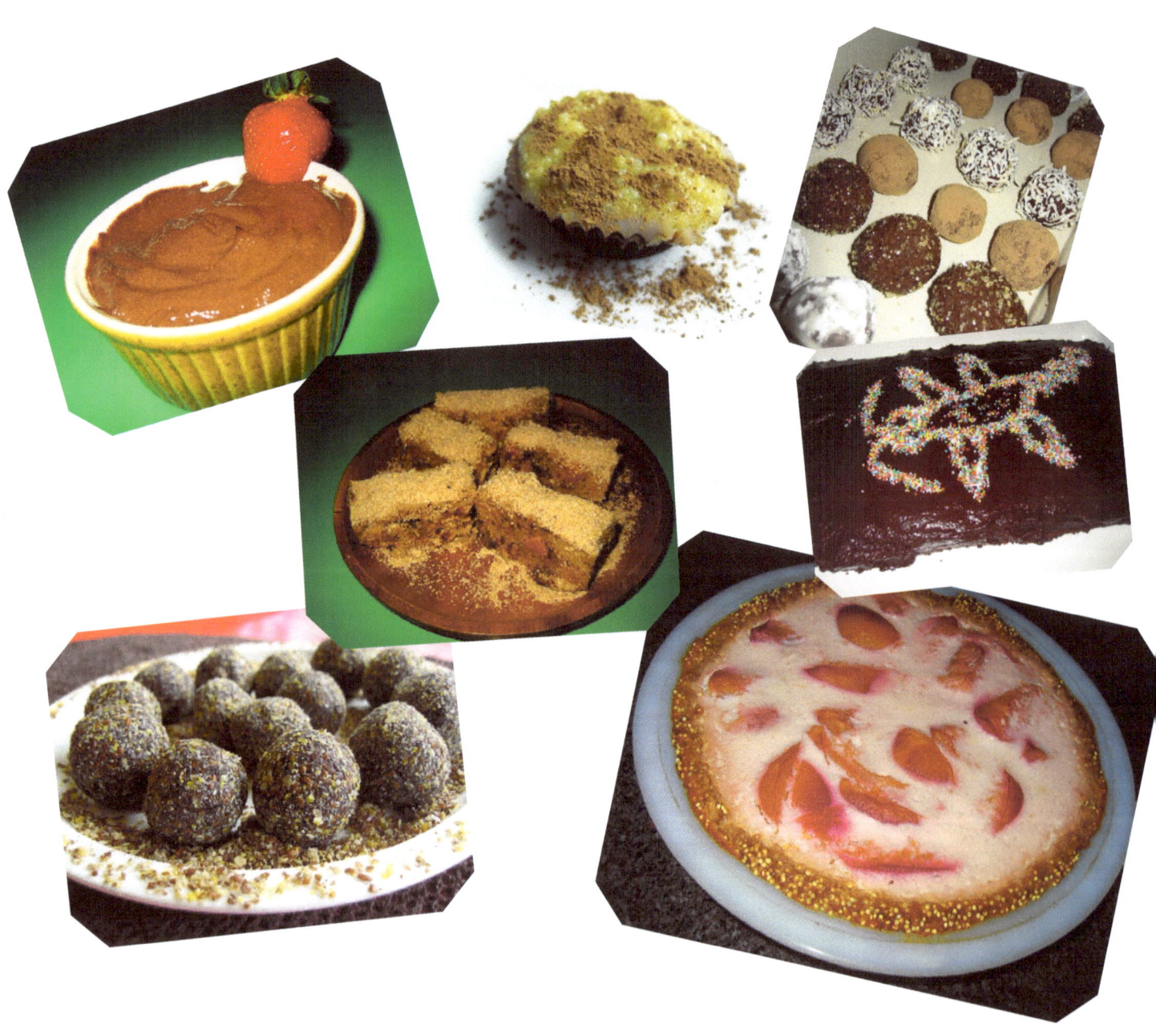

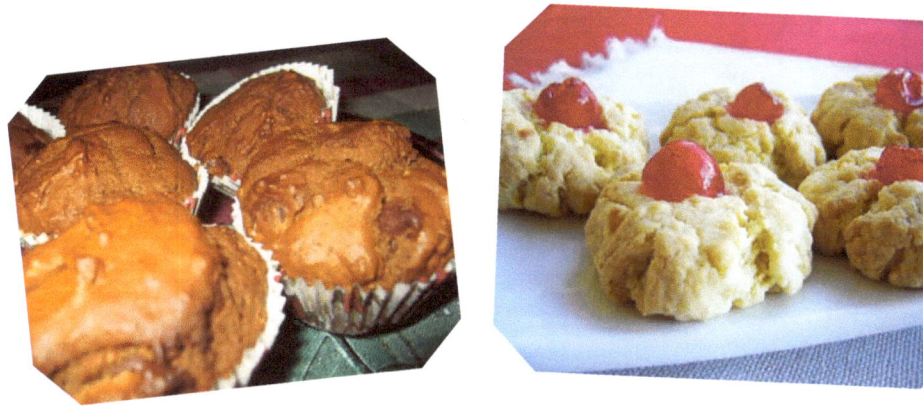

Others include my decadent chocolate cake, cupcakes and truffles, cherry shortbread as well as some more healthier detox recipes including nectarine and tofu pie, polenta health slice, carob and date balls and raw cashew cream with raw chocolate.

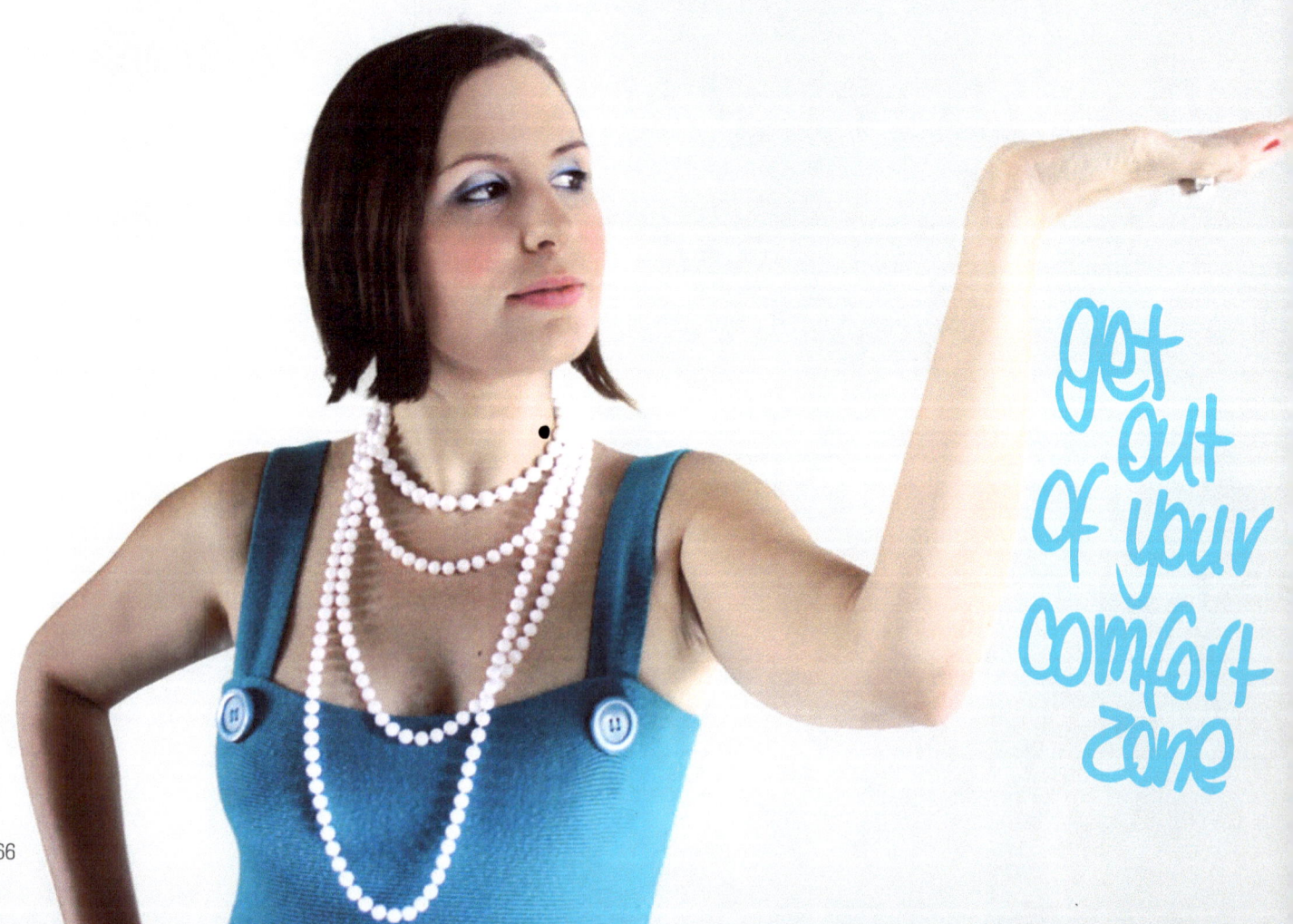

There are so many alternatives to the boring mainstream diet, I hope I have inspired you with my vegan meals and you have some new ideas of what to cook. The Internet is a great source for all vegan options. Whatever your favourite dish, do a search to find the vegan version. Be creative and versatile with your cooking. Think outside the square, shop for your food products at different places, frequent farmers markets, Chinese and Indian supermarkets to expand your horizons. Remember to do your research, eat all of the colours of the rainbow in your diet and consume all of the vegan staples. Good luck!

Viva la Vegan! started to promote Leigh-Chantelle's Recipe Calendars in 2005 and has since grown to be an interactive community for vegans focusing on positive education, information and vegan outreach. Through the vivalavegan.net website, Leigh-Chantelle's focus is on educating people to alternative lifestyle choices, proving that via compassion we can heal ourselves and each other.

vivalavegan.net focuses on easy to prepare recipes, blogs, articles and podcasts; interactive forum, informative and how-to videos, interviews with inspiring vegans, vegan mentoring and much more.

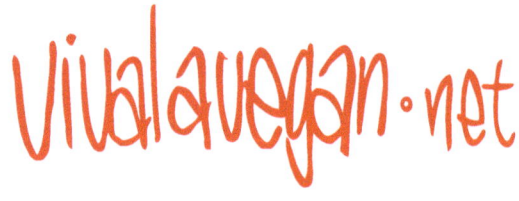

About the Author

Leigh-Chantelle lives mostly in sunny Brisbane, Australia where she runs the online vegan community vivalavegan.net, the not-for-profit environmental awareness Green Earth Group, as well as coordinates Online Etiquette Education and Social Media Marketing with Epicentre Equilibrium. Leigh-Chantelle believes in the rights of all beings, networking, surrounding herself with people on the same life path as her and she is a bit obsessed with quinoa.

Leigh-Chantelle is an accredited Naturopath, Nutritionist and Western Herbalist who combines her passion for vegan health along with her natural therapies and healing skills. Leigh-Chantelle has released three *Viva la Vegan!* recipe calendars, a plant-based Detox Diet e-book as well as re-released her recipe calendars as recycled recipe cards. Over the past 15 years since Leigh-Chantelle has been a vegan she has been involved as a sponsor, performer, speaker, emcee and stallholder for various animal rights, vegan, vegetarian, environmental and cruelty-free fundraisers, forums, conferences, festivals and events throughout Australia and internationally.

Leigh-Chantelle is available for select speaking engagements, seminars, panel discussions and readings on the following:

- Veganism, Animal Rights and Activism
- Staging Effective Events, Engaging Volunteers and Team Work
- Online Etiquette, Social Media Marketing and Online Skills

To enquire about a possible appearance, please contact email@vivalavegan.net

You can find Leigh-Chantelle, Viva la Vegan!, Green Earth Group and Epicentre Equilibrium on

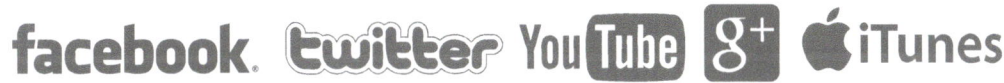

www.ingramcontent.com/pod-product-compliance
Lightning Source LLC
Chambersburg PA
CBHW061402090426
42743CB00003B/120